The
ARTHRITIS
SOLUTION

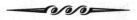

About the Authors

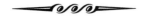

Joseph Kandel, M.D., is the founder and medical director of the Neurology Center of Naples in Naples, Florida, and cofounder of the Gulfcoast Spine Institute. He is also an associate clinical professor at Wright State University School of Medicine. An avid student since his youth, he attended Ohio State University as a Batelle Scholar, obtaining a double major B.S. in zoology and a B.S. in psychology, both with honors. Kandel graduated from Wright State University School of Medicine in Dayton, Ohio, in 1985, where he was president of his freshman medical school class. He completed his residency at the University of California Irvine Medical Center.

Kandel is a popular public speaker and has been published in such prestigious medical journals as *Neurology, Vital Signs,* and *American Zoologist.*

He lives in Naples with his wife and their three children.

David Sudderth, M.D., is the senior partner at the Neurology Center of Naples and is cofounder of the Gulfcoast Spine Institute in Naples, Florida.

He graduated from medical school at the University of Copenhagen in 1984 and completed his residency at the Medical College of Wisconsin and Emory University. Dr. Sudderth accomplished a one-year fellowship in nerve and muscle disorders at Emory University in 1988.

An in-demand lecturer, Sudderth speaks frequently on medical topics. He also produced the popular video *Spinal Tips* and has published in *Neurology* and *Ugeskrift For Laeger.*

An avid computer fan, Dr. Sudderth can often be found perusing the Internet and other computer services, adding to his extensive knowledge of neurological issues and problems.

The
ARTHRITIS SOLUTION

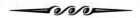

Joseph Kandel, M.D.
and
David B. Sudderth, M.D.

PRIMA PUBLISHING

Warning—Disclaimer

Prima Publishing has designed this book to provide information in regard to the subject matter covered. It is sold with the understanding that the publisher and the author are not liable for the misconception or misuse of information provided. Every effort has been made to make this book as complete and as accurate as possible. The purpose of this book is to educate. The author and Prima Publishing shall have neither liability nor responsibility to any person or entity with respect to any loss, damage, or injury caused or alleged to be caused directly or indirectly by the information contained in this book. The information presented herein is in no way intended as a substitute for medical counseling.

Names have been changed to protect the privacy of patients.

Library of Congress Cataloging-in-Publication Data
Kandel, Joseph.
    The arthritis solution / Joseph Kandel and David B. Sudderth.
        p. cm.
    Includes bibliographical references and index.
    ISBN 0-7615-1172-5
        1. Osteoarthritis—Popular works.   I. Sudderth, David B.
    II. Title.
    RC931.O67K96   1997
    616.7'223—dc21   97-13641
                                                                      CIP

97 98 99 HH 10 9 8 7 6 5 4 3 2 1
Printed in the United States of America

All products mentioned in this book are trademarks of their respective companies.

How to Order

Single copies may be ordered from Prima Publishing, P.O. Box 1260, Rocklin, CA 95677; telephone (916) 632-4400. Quantity discounts are also available. On your letterhead, include information concerning the intended use of the books and the number of books you wish to purchase.

Visit us online at http://www.primapublishing.com

To my wife, Merrylee, for all of your patience, kindness, love, and warmth—I thank you. Your constant support makes everything possible.

—JOSEPH KANDEL

For Mai Lea

—DAVID B. SUDDERTH

Contents

Preface

A year ago, Marie had severe arthritis, and if she could have seen into the future with a crystal ball, she would have been amazed. After following a combination of medications, special magnets, and a weight loss program, Marie now leads an active, normal life. No wheelchairs or canes for her!

Marie is only one of hundreds of success stories we've had of people with agonizing arthritis who were told by other doctors that they had to "learn to live with it." Why in the world should you learn to live with the pain and disability of arthritis if you don't have to? Why should you give up your life? Why should you risk depression and further pain and suffering? Our rousing answer to you is that you should definitely NOT live with it. You don't have to.

Maybe you and even your doctor don't know this: arthritis is not a prison sentence, and you're not starting on a course of ever-increasing pain. Instead, it is very possible today to resume a normal life, using a combination of traditional treatments, alternative options, and actions that you can take yourself.

We have written this book to send you the news bulletins you need on the latest medicines, procedures, and options. We explain to you what arthritis is and what illnesses many people (and sometimes doctors) confuse with it. We talk about the most effective medicines on the market today and we also discuss a variety of natural "medicines" that work to make you feel better.

We discuss a broad array of treatments that help people with arthritis, from massage to heat packs to mud baths to the special magnets that helped Marie so much. We've spent years learning everything we can about alleviating the pain of arthritis, and we've learned what works—and what doesn't.

Some of the actions you can take may not seem medical, such as losing weight. Every doctor you've ever met has probably hounded you about weight loss. We have some easy and fun exercises for you to try. As well, you'll learn about the latest weight loss medication, Redux.

We also talk about the future. Cloning human cells is a technique that is already here now. Some doctors are genetically reengineering cells—actually taking them out, tagging them with an arthritis-resistant DNA, and then putting them back into the person. We're talking cure here. Such treatments are still a few years from common usage, but they're on their way.

Pain Relief Is Not a One-Step, Immediate Process

Millions of Americans would like a quick fix or an instant cure for arthritis. Take a few pills, and your arthritis and pain are gone. This is the primary appeal of books such as *The Arthritis Cure* by Jason Theodosakis, M.D., a book that touts glucosamine sulfate and chondroitin sulfate as substances that, combined, "can halt, reverse, and may even *cure* osteoarthritis." We know that you can gain pain relief from your arthritis, but it's usually more involved than popping a few pills.

When a Cure Is Not a Cure

Does *The Arthritis Cure* really deliver a "cure" for arthritis? Not in the sense that most of us think of the word *cure*. Most people believe that a cure means first, you have an illness, then—after some sort of intervention—the illness is gone. What Dr. Theodosakis does, however, is redefine the word *cure* to mean "partial or complete relief of symptoms." He also states that nothing in the book is "intended to suggest that the use of the recommended supplements will fully eradicate osteoarthritis."

Are the over-the-counter products glucosamine sulfate and chondroitin sulfate of any value at all? In this book, we look at the pros and cons of this much-discussed combination treatment for treating arthritis and other joint pain syndromes (Chapter 6). We also consider a broad array of other treatments that can ease, and in some cases radically reduce, the pain and problems associated with arthritis (Chapters 4 and 5).

The Combination Lock of Arthritis Relief

Just because we can̓t immediately cure arthritis today does *not* mean there isn̓t much that we—and you—can do now. There is a lot you can do and a lot you can ask your doctor to do. We offer practical and immediately usable suggestions in this book. We see the path to chronic arthritis pain relief as a combination lock; and to achieve pain relief, you need to dial in the right combination of treatments for you.

Successful treatment can also be viewed as a jigsaw puzzle. You need all the pieces to get a complete picture.

Find What Works for You

Our goal here is to present you with various pieces of the puzzle, so you and your doctor will be able to put together your own picture of pain relief. The pieces may comprise traditional medication, dietary changes, weight loss, exercise, massage, magnets, or any of more than two dozen other treatments. The point is, arthritis pain relief is almost invariably achieved by a combination of actions. Design the right arthritis solution for *you*!

The important thing is, don't let anyone, including your doctor, put you up on the shelf. Take charge of your life. Marie did, and so have hundreds of our other patients. Read this book and follow our advice. And write to us and let us know how you're doing. We care. What works for you might work for someone else, and we'd like to hear about it.

Doctors Kandel and Sudderth
Attn: Kari DiBene
670 Goodlette Road, North
Naples, FL 34102

Acknowledgments

Thank you to Chris Adamec for her keen insight, her constructive comments and criticisms, and her biting humor throughout the preparation of this text.

And to the entire staff at Neuroscience and Spine Associates—thank you for putting up with us during the writing of this book.

1

Introduction:
What Is Osteoarthritis?

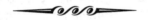

Arthritis is an inflammatory disease affecting the joints, which can cause agonizing pain. Osteoarthritis has been called a degenerative disease and is even called "degenerative joint disease" (for simplicity, we'll call the illness "arthritis" in most of the book). Arthritis is not a modern ailment. In fact, arthritis has been a problem for people worldwide since before recorded time. At least fourteen ancient Roman emperors knew the pain of arthritis. And you can go all the way back to prehistoric time and see evidence of arthritis: archaeologists have found arthritis in the bones of cave dwellers. If you suffer from arthritis, you have plenty of company—about 41 million people in the United States alone.

The good news is that you and your fellow men and women with arthritis are now entering not only the chronological new millennium but also a new millennium of treatments, medications, and strategies to beat this problem into submission. Some of the "new" treatments, such as magnetic therapy, special diets, and other techniques, were popular many years ago, some even thousands of years ago.

This book will describe the latest and greatest treatments, medicines, devices, and other curative measures to help you return to an active and healthy life. We'll talk about what arthritis is and how it is diagnosed. We'll describe other illnesses that are sometimes confused with arthritis. Most important, this book will give you practical and immediately usable advice on what you can do about this illness, including using traditional therapies and medications as well as nontraditional treatments, such as magnetic therapy, vitamin therapy, biofeedback, and much more. There are definitely many actions that you, in collaboration with your doctor, can take to improve your arthritis problem, to cut back (or eliminate) the pain, and to resume a healthy and active life.

First, let's get a handle on this disease.

The Human Joint

Let's consider the anatomy and physiology of a normal joint. We will talk about the basic features of joints that are typically affected by osteoarthritis.

A joint is merely a structure that allows two objects to move independently to some degree. A door hinge is a simple mechanical example, but it's obviously not composed of living, breathing tissue. The design specifications for human joints are very complex.

Joint surfaces are formed by a thick layer of cartilage resting on bone. This cartilaginous material is called the articular surface (articulation means joint). There are no blood vessels in the cartilage (blood vessels supply living tissue with essential nutrients and transport waste products to other sites in the body, where they can ultimately be eliminated). The cartilage also has no nerve endings, which is why, even though healthy joint surfaces support massive weight, no pain is reported to the brain.

If you look at cartilage microscopically, you can see that it is comprised of two features: (1) the *chondrocyte* and (2) the ground substance, called the *extracellular matrix*. The ground substance is composed primarily of water (one of the earliest changes seen in arthritis is the loss of water) and is a very complex three-dimensional ray of interlocking strands of collagen.

Collagen is a very tough protein that prevents major distortions of the ground substance when normal pressure is applied to joint surfaces. Attached to and covering this framework of collagen fibers are the *proteoglycans* and *hyaluronic acid* (aggrecan). These are very large molecules that maintain the content and direct the flow of fluid circulating throughout the joint surface.

When pressure is applied to the joints, the cartilaginous structures are compressed. As movement stops or the body relaxes, the cartilage can reexpand. This compression and relaxation allows nutrient-bearing fluid to circulate freely in the joint. This fluid is formed by the *synovial membrane,* which is a very thin structure lining the joint capsule much like a sleeve or a tube. Thus, when we are moving, we are actually feeding our joints. Conversely, when we stop moving, we are starving our joints.

The joint must be able to withstand hundreds of pounds of force for long periods of time, without causing pain. The surfaces of the joint must also be able to move quite freely against each other. This is accomplished in part by the synovial fluid, which coats the joint surfaces and allows movement with only a tiny amount of friction.

Closely related to joints are *tendons* and *bursae.* A tendon is a tough structure that attaches muscle to bone. The lubricating system of tendons is similar to that of joints. Bursa are small, collapsed structures that allow skin and subcutaneous tissue to move freely over joints. They can be compared to a collapsed balloon, with a thin film of water allowing opposing surfaces of the balloon to move freely. Both tendons and bursae are involved in the arthritic process and can be potent pain generators.

What Goes Wrong?

We have to say from the outset that the cause of osteoarthritis remains unknown. That does not mean we know nothing or that medical theories tell us nothing. The condition of arthritis appears to be a problem of maintenance. Let's compare it to the maintenance of a well-functioning factory. A factory needs raw materials, and its waste products need to be eliminated. Proper mixing, finishing, and repairing are all well-known maintenance issues.

This maintenance process applies to your joints. Raw materials must be provided to the chondrocytes, which in turn provide the materials for the ground substance. The chondrocytes produce not only the ground substance but also enzymes, which help protect the ground substance. This is a necessary part of replacing "worn-out tissue."

We don't know what sets off the cascade leading to the arthritic process. At any rate, the joint loses water, and in the early stages there can be some thickening of the cartilage, which ultimately softens due to the loss of fluid in the ground substance.

Because of the change in consistency of the cartilage, small clefts develop in the cartilage. As these clefts deepen, they extend fully to the bone. The chondrocytes proliferate in a futile attempt to shore up the deteriorating cartilage.

Changes are soon seen in the bone underneath the cartilage. As the cartilage is braided, dense calcification occurs on the surface of the bone, which may begin to look like ivory (eburnation). Proliferation of bone and cartilage leads to bone spurs (osteophytes). Bone spurs change the configuration of the joints and can lead to major deformity.

Accompanying these changes is a thickening and often some inflammation in the synovial fluid lining the joint capsules. All these processes lead not only to deformation of the joint but also to varying degrees of loss of normal range of motion. The joint capsule also thickens, which further limits movement.

Since the joints are no longer able to move properly, the muscles that move the joint shrink and become weaker, leading to even greater instability of the joint. Because of this loss of motion and inability to exercise in general, the arthritic process is a self-sustaining one.

The Pain

We mentioned that there are no nerve fibers in the joint cartilage. So where does all the pain come from? There are many pain-sensitive structures. The synovial membrane often becomes inflamed, a process that leads to production of nerve-irritating chemicals. The bone under the cartilage is extremely sensitive to pain, and there can even be small fractures in this portion of the bone. Bone spurs will stretch the *periosteum* (the exquisitely pain-sensitive lining of bones), leading to severe pain. The ligaments, which are the fiber structures attaching bone to bone, can also be stretched, which can be tremendously painful. The joint capsule can be inflamed and stretched, and muscles surrounding this painful mass often will contract involuntarily (spasm) to reduce the very painful motion of the joint.

Progressive joint deterioration can also cause other painful symptoms that may not be immediately associated with arthritis. For example, the deterioration could lead to a pinched nerve in the neck or in the low back. Wrist arthritis and tendinitis can lead to carpal tunnel syndrome (a compressed nerve at the wrist), leading to nerve pain in the hand as well as numbness, muscle weakness, and loss of function of the affected hand. Spinal nerves can also be involved in this nightmarish process. Deterioration can cause pinched nerves and even spinal cord damage. Severe headaches may be caused by arthritis-related tissue proliferation in the small joints at the upper portion of the spine.

Who Gets Arthritis?

Arthritis typically affects people who are over forty years of age; it is especially a problem for people in their sixties and seventies. Osteoarthritis is the most common cause of disability in the industrial world. In this country alone, approximately $55 billion per year is lost to the economy as a consequence of lost work days, medication, and other treatments. This represents almost 1 percent of the United States gross domestic product (GDP). Don't be one of those statistics—take the actions that we recommend in this book!

Up to about age fifty-five, arthritis is an equal opportunity disability, and the disease affects the same joints in men and women. After age fifty-five, hip arthritis is somewhat more common in men, while arthritis of the hands and knees are more common in women. The spectrum of this disorder can vary widely from a minor morning ache to total invalidism.

Risk Factors

A risk factor is an internal or external influence that appears to be related to a given disease, and there are several types of risk factors for arthritis, including metabolic, genetic, mechanical, and age-related. The most potent risk factor for arthritis is clearly age. Another risk factor is your sex: women are more prone to experience some forms of arthritis, while men have to deal with others. Age and sex could combine to be strong risk factors. In one study of females, only 2 percent of the women under the age of forty-five had any suggestion of osteoarthritis; after the age of sixty-five, the incidence was nearly 70 percent.

Your own genetic structure can also determine whether you ultimately become arthritic. This is particularly true of the earlier onset types of this disorder.

Another risk factor for arthritis is if you incur an injury to your joints, either because of a major trauma or because of repetitive joint use. As a result, athletes are at risk for arthritis at a relatively young age. Boxers tend to develop arthritic disease in their hands, while ballet dancers tend to experience ankle arthritis as a common consequence of their craft.

It's also true that bone fractures involving joints typically lead to arthritis. Studies on textile workers have demonstrated that laborers tend to get arthritis, particularly in the joints involved repetitively in their specific task. This is also true of jackhammer operators and coal miners, among others.

Weight Is Clearly a Factor   It's fairly obvious that being overweight can cause or exacerbate arthritis; this has been demonstrated recently by investigators. This appears to be particularly true of the knee joints and more for women than for men.

Obesity is a "modifiable" risk factor: while we can't change our genes or how old we are, we can certainly change the size of our waistlines. Add twenty or thirty—or more—pounds on an already strained system, and ouch! Conversely, losing those pounds and freeing up your joints can help considerably. Admittedly, though, losing weight can be difficult for many people. See the latest medication and therapy advice on how to lose weight in Chapter 8.

Smoking May Be a Factor   There is also some controversy about whether smoking is a direct risk factor for arthritis. We believe that it is. Certainly, it is a risk factor for at least one type of spine disorder: degenerative disc disease. Smoking is also associated with an inactive lifestyle and muscle weakness, both of which are risk factors for progression of osteoarthritis.

Other Risk Factors   As we stated earlier, a previous injury to a joint can cause arthritis. Gout and other inflammatory processes (which we describe in Chapter 2) can cause this type of injury, which, in turn, can lead to arthritis. A hemorrhage into a joint can cause severe inflammation, leading to arthritis. An extreme example of a joint hemorrhage is the joint deformities seen in people with hemophilia.

Unrecognized and therefore usually quite subtle abnormalities of joint alignment that you may have been born with can also lead to future arthritis. We've been doing formal screenings of infants for many years, and by doing so, we have treated the problem immediately and reduced the cases of adult osteoarthritis in the region.

Living with Arthritis

For most people, arthritis equals pain, and this pain can be quite severe. Typically, the pain is described as a deep aching sensation and is aggravated by movement. Some relief comes with rest, especially in the early stages of arthritis. As the condition worsens, pain at night may become quite severe, impairing sleep. A painful stiffness in the morning becomes the sufferer's permanent wake-up call. The stiffness can also occur after a person has been inactive, for example, after sitting in a movie or after a meal.

As individuals become increasingly affected by their disease, they can become essentially immobile. Often, wracked by pain for years, these individuals become very depressed and are essentially unable to exercise.

Exercise Is Critically Important

Science has proven beyond any doubt that if you do not exercise, you will age in dog years. The list of consequences of not exercising regularly include, but are not limited to, the following:

- Worsened arthritis
- Elevated blood pressure
- Elevated blood sugar and cholesterol

- Depression and insomnia
- Increased risk for infections and some types of cancer because of immune compromise
- Increased risk for coronary artery disease and stroke
- Increased risk of falls with severe injury, such as bone fractures or intracranial hemorrhage
- Obesity
- Circulatory failure in the limbs

Be sure to read Chapter 8 for important new information on healthful lifestyles and avoiding depression.

Now that you have some basic information under your belt about arthritis, let's move on to our next chapter and the many different illnesses that can be (and are) confused with arthritis.

2

If It's Not Arthritis, What Else Could It Be?

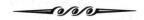

If you're suffering from pain that seems to come from one or more of your joints, you might hear your father, sister, or best friend tell you that this is just the way that he or she feels, too: it's arthritis. Continue loving your family and friends, and thank them for their information—then ask your doctor to help you find the cause of your problem. There are many other illnesses that have arthritis-like symptoms, and you need to know what the real problem is. If you have an illness that is not arthritis, you may need treatment that is very different from what a person with arthritis would need.

When you see your doctor about the joint pain you're experiencing, he or she will review your medical history (or take your history, if the doctor is new to you) and then examine you. The doctor may order tests as well. Then the doctor will consider a variety of medical problems that you may have: this is called a "differential diagnosis," because the doctor is ruling out (or in) illnesses that seem to fit your problem pattern. This chapter covers illnesses that are most like and are most likely to be confused with osteoarthritis.

Rheumatoid Arthritis

Rheumatoid arthritis is another arthritic condition, and it is the one that nondoctors confuse most frequently with osteoarthritis. It can be a very severe disease that affects not only joints but also many other organ systems. Approximately 1 percent of the population suffers from rheumatoid arthritis. It is more common in women; the female to male ratio is approximately 3 to 1. The illness usually appears when the person is in his or her forties. It is a strongly genetic condition, although identical twins do not always both have this disease, so some environmental factors must also play a role in its development.

The disease apparently begins in the synovial membrane, where intense inflammation occurs and then spreads to the cartilage. Cartilage and bone become eroded, and joints often become very deformed. Rheumatoid arthritis is considered to be one of the autoimmune diseases, which means the body creates antibodies (disease-fighting proteins) but they are misdirected toward the body of the person rather than at bacteria or illness.

The problem can harm many other parts of the body in addition to the joints. Rheumatoid arthritis can lead to serious diseases of the skin, lungs, heart, and arteries. It can even cause a lethal condition, pericarditis, which is inflammation and fluid collection surrounding the heart. It can also affect the spinal cord.

The diagnosis of rheumatoid arthritis is primarily based on the patient's history and physical examination. The patient typically has a symmetrical (same on both sides) inflammation of the small and large joints in the arms and legs. Small knots under the skin (subcutaneous nodules) also help the doctor make the diagnosis. Another symptom is the presence of an abnormal antibody in the blood, known as rheumatoid factor. This refers to abnormal cells in the synovial fluid. X-rays also can confirm these findings.

Pain control and reduction of inflammation is the primary emphasis in treating rheumatoid arthritis. A person may also need physical therapy. Sometimes joint replacements are required. Nonsteroidal anti-inflammatory drugs (NSAIDs) are often used to treat rheumatoid arthritis. These medications don't prevent progressive joint destruction, but they can help somewhat with the problems of inflammation and pain control. (For more information on NSAIDs and other medications, see Chapter 4.) Steroids are another form of medication used to treat this disorder. The problem with steroids is that they can cause osteoporosis, and they have other side effects.

Good news on the horizon: a new category of medication, "biological response modifiers," should be available for treating this disease in the near future. This medication would be administered by injection and would block the inflammation cascade at the joint level. These new, genetically engineered agents may dramatically change the treatment of this destructive disorder.

Systemic Lupus Erythematosus (Lupus)

Like rheumatoid arthritis, systemic lupus erythematosus can be a devastating illness. It affects not only the joints but also many other tissues, and it can be fatal. Most people with this illness are females in their twenties and thirties, and it is somewhat more common in African-American women.

The most obvious symptom of lupus is a "butterfly" rash over the bridge of the nose, chin, and cheeks, in the general form of a butterfly. Essentially all organ systems, including the central nervous system, can be affected by this disorder. The joints of the hands and feet as well as of the wrists and knees are primarily affected. Severe joint deformities are fairly uncommon with this disease. Use of chronic steroids can lead to severe muscle and bone weakness.

If the brain is affected, seizures, dementia, and even psychosis can occur. As with rheumatoid arthritis, lupus appears to be an autoimmune disease. Patients nearly always have profound fatigue and joint and muscle pain, and they may also have intermittent arthritis. Various treatments exist, ranging from medications, steroids, and chemotherapy to exercise, diet, and lifestyle modifications.

Systemic Sclerosis (Scleroderma)

Scleroderma is another multiorgan disorder in which there is an increased amount of tough connective tissue (fibrosis) in the skin, abdominal organs, blood vessels, heart, lungs, and kidneys. Patients with this illness can have abnormal blood vessels in the skin and abnormal calcification in many organs, and they may also suffer major problems with the esophagus, leading to difficulty swallowing.

In the early stages of the disease, the fingers and hands are swollen, and the face and legs may also swell. This swelling tends to become quite firm. Over half the patients with this disorder complain of pain, stiffness, and swelling in the fingers and both knees symmetrically. They may also develop symptoms of carpal tunnel syndrome. Muscle weakness is often a feature of this disorder. Blood testing often reveals a specific, abnormal antibody in this disease.

The Raynaud's phenomenon is a common feature of this disorder. In this case, the patient first experiences "puffiness" in the fingers. When exposed to cold, blood vessels in the fingers and even tip of the nose and ear lobes suddenly constrict (close). At first these areas become very white, and then they turn blue. Eventually, the blue gives way to a redness as the blood returns to the region.

Drug treatment for this disorder is quite unsatisfactory and is typically fraught with major side effects. Interestingly, the Raynaud's phenomenon described above can often be improved by biofeedback training, which is discussed in Chapter 5.

Dermatomyositis and Polymyositis

Polymyositis is a disease that usually involves the large muscles by the hips and buttocks as well as the large muscles in the shoulder area. This disorder appears to be an autoimmune disease. This condition is frequently associated with a characteristic skin rash: a lilac-colored rash on the eyelids, bridge of the nose, and cheeks, which can also occur in the nail beds and on the hands. When the rash is present, the condition is called dermatomyositis.

Patients can have serious weakness and can even have difficulty swallowing and breathing. Severe pain is present in only 10 percent of these patients and primarily occurs in the buttocks, thighs, and the lower portion of the legs, especially the calves. A particularly serious variation of this disease involves the heart muscle and can be fatal.

The illness can develop suddenly or over a period of months. In approximately 10 percent of the cases, sufferers develop a malignancy. In about one-third of the cases, other connective tissue disorders, such as rheumatoid arthritis, mixed connective tissue disease, scleroderma, or lupus also are present. Treatment is usually primarily steroid-based.

Mixed Connective Tissue Disease

Mixed connective tissue disease (MCTD) is a syndrome that typically occurs in the late thirties, and approximately 80 percent of the patients are women. Most patients have swollen joints of the hands, making the fingers resemble sausages. Various skin rashes may occur. This is a form of arthritis, although it is not osteoarthritis. It may resemble mild cases of rheumatoid arthritis.

Mild muscle weakness occurs with MCTD, and patients also often have a malfunctioning esophagus. Severe lung disease often complicates this disorder. Steroids are often used in treating this disease.

Sjogren's Syndrome

This is another example of an autoimmune disorder, and it is a form of arthritis. With Sjogren's syndrome, the white blood cells infiltrate the tear and salivary glands, resulting in extreme dryness of the eyes and mouth. This disease affects primarily middle-aged women (with a 9 to 1 ratio of women to men).

Approximately one-third of these patients will have other symptoms, such as fatigue, muscle pain, and pain in multiple joints. The arthritis involvement with this disorder is rarely of a debilitating or destructive nature.

No treatment of any type has been shown to alter the course of Sjogren's syndrome. Instead, treatment is directed toward preventing injuries related to the dryness of the eyes, such as corneal ulceration.

Ankylosing Spondylitis

Ankylosing spondylitis is an inflammatory disease primarily affecting the spine, although in rare cases, the joints of the arms and legs are affected. Men have this disease three times more frequently than women, and symptoms usually appear in patients in their teens or twenties.

This disorder is highly associated (90 percent) with a specific gene (HLA-B27). Severe low back pain is usually the characteristic feature of ankylosing spondylitis. Significant joint deterioration occurs with this illness; ultimately, the joint is completely obliterated. Characteristic x-ray findings are generally present in this disorder.

Elsewhere in the spine, doctors find involvement of the intervertebral disc and cartilage. Sometimes inflammation of the eyes also occurs, and there is occasionally some involvement of the great blood vessels. This disease is painful, and the patient's posture becomes increasingly stooped.

Arthritis affecting the hips and shoulder joints may occur in approximately one-third of these individuals, while joints of the elbows, hands, wrists, knees, and feet are usually spared. As the disease progresses, the spine becomes increasingly rigid and fractures may occur. If the fractures involve the upper portion of the neck, it can lead to complete paralysis.

Even though this is a severe and progressive disease, most individuals with this disorder are able to continue working, and this disorder does not usually shorten the individual's life. Treatment is primarily symptomatic and commonly involves nonsteroidal anti-inflammatory drugs (NSAIDs). Exercise therapy may also slow the progression of the rigidity. Total hip replacement may be necessary and often results in an enormous improvement in the patient's overall status, including mobility as well as pain relief.

Behcet's Syndrome

Behcet's syndrome is a fairly rare disease that usually involves severe ulcerations of the mouth. Other symptoms include recurrent sores about the genitals and various other sites, including the skin and eyes. Arthritic involvement can occur as well and primarily affects ankles and knee joints; however, it is usually not deforming. Unlike most other diseases, this illness often diminishes with age.

Steroids are often a prominent treatment of this disorder. Involvement of the eyes can lead to rapidly progressive blindness.

Reiter's Syndrome (Reactive Arthritis)

Reiter's syndrome is an inflammatory condition in which arthritis may be a very severe feature. The arthritis usually involves the large weight-bearing joints, especially the knees and ankles. Other features of this disorder include inflammation of the urethra or the bladder and inflammation of the eye, and there can also be lesions affecting the mucus membranes of the mouth and skin.

The gene HLA-B27, previously mentioned in connection with ankylosing spondylitis, is present in 80 percent of white patients with this disorder. Reiter's syndrome is also called "reactive arthritis" because it comes in the wake of an infection such as gastroenteritis or a sexually transmitted disease such as a chlamydial infection.

The arthritic involvement can be very painful, and often the patient has severely swollen and very hot joints. Recurrences of this disorder are common and can even be permanent—this is especially true of joint involvement. Nonsteroidal anti-inflammatory drugs (NSAIDs) are frequently used in this disorder. Antibiotics also appear to play a role in treatment of this disorder and in reducing the likelihood of relapse.

Polymyalgia Rheumatica (PMR) and Giant Cell Arteritis (Temporal Arteritis)

These two illnesses are probably a spectrum of one disease. The patients who develop these disorders are usually over fifty years of age and have some blood serologies in common.

Polymyalgia rheumatica is diagnosed based on the patient's symptoms and physical examination. Usually patients suffer from fatigue; fluctuating fever and weight loss may also occur. Pain and stiffness in the shoulder and pelvic girdle area are the usual complaints. Patients may have difficulty holding their arms above their shoulders and find getting dressed and combing their hair painful. They may also have discomfort in the knees and wrists. Anemia is also possible.

Patients typically respond very well to low-dose steroids, usually 10 to 20 mg per day. Often the response to therapy is very rapid. Once a therapeutic approach is obtained, typically the drug is slowly withdrawn. Treatment usually lasts six to twenty-four months.

Giant cell arteritis involves the medium and large arteries. The temporal artery, a fairly large artery that supplies the scalp, is often involved. This is a nonessential artery and can easily be removed by a surgeon and examined under the microscope, subsequently leading to a diagnosis of this disorder. Approximately half of these patients will have polymyalgia rheumatica as well. This disease is much more serious than polymyalgia rheumatica, because it can involve arteries of the cranium and eyes and can lead to blindness.

Patients usually suffer severe head pain and many also have pain in the jaw, which is made worse by speaking or chewing. This disease responds very well to fairly high doses of steroids, usually in the range of 60 mg per day. After symptomatic relief is obtained in about six to eight weeks, the drug can be gradually withdrawn.

Patients with this disorder typically have an elevated ESR (erythrocyte sedimentation rate), which is a very nonspecific measure of immune response.

Gouty Arthritis

Gout is a disease of high levels of uric acid. Ninety percent of patients with this disorder are male, and most are over the age of thirty. There is also a very high hereditary component to this disorder. When women are stricken with gout, it usually occurs after menopause.

The disease appears to be related to the crystallization of uric acid in the joints. This leads to a severe inflammatory reaction. The crystallization of uric acid can also lead to knots in other tissues.

The onset is sudden and extremely acute and usually occurs at night (a painful way to be awakened). Gout generally involves one joint, usually the base of the big toe. The toe may be very swollen—even touching this joint is extremely painful. It's impossible for the toe to bear any weight during an acute attack of gouty arthritis. Other affected areas can include the feet, ankles, and knees. Occasionally more than one joint may be involved in an attack. Fever may also occur.

Gout responds very well to nonsteroidal anti-inflammatory drugs (NSAIDs) and to colchicine. The ancient Romans used colchicine to treat gout, and the first known use was by a fifth-century physician, Jacob Psychristus, nearly 1,500 years ago!

Chondrocalcinosis and Pseudogout

Chondrocalcinosis implies the presence of calcium salts in the cartilage of joints. It is often demonstrated on x-rays. This type of disorder is usually genetic and can be seen with other diseases, such as thyroid disorders and diabetes.

Pseudogout is a disease usually affecting individuals over the age of sixty; it typically reoccurs regularly and comes on suddenly with great severity. Only rarely is arthritic involvement chronic. Typically the joints are very tender and warm and the fluid obtained from the joint shows a specific type of crystal, calcium pyrophosphate.

Therapies often include heat and ice treatment, standard combination physical therapy, and various medications. The different types of "traditional" physical therapies are discussed in Chapter 7.

Psoriasis

Psoriasis is a common dermatologic condition that may affect up to two-thirds of the population. This disease is an inflammatory reaction and involves varying sizes of red plaque eruptions that are sharply different from the surrounding skin. Often there is a flaking, silvery material over the lesions, which may or may not itch. Often the elbows, knees, and scalp are affected, and there may also be severe deformities of the nails. A wide spectrum of arthritic problems can arise in patients with psoriasis. Occasionally, the arthritis is severe and leads to fairly rapid destruction of the joints involved. The arthritic component of psoriasis is usually limited to the spine. Chemotherapeutic agents, such as methotrexate, are commonly used in this disorder as well as various local medications such as steroids.

Paget's Disease of Bone (Osteitis Deformans)

Deep bone pain is usually the first symptom of this disorder. Paget's disease appears to be related to excessive bone destruction, leading to significant deformities in the bones. Often the characteristic bony regrowth is visible in an x-ray examination. The disease leads to an enlargement of the head, which can interfere with the auditory canal and cause deafness. The tibia (large bone in the calf) also becomes bowed outward, and the midportion of the spine becomes increasingly curved forward. Fractures of these abnormal bones can occur even when the trauma is fairly mild. Headaches frequently accompany this disorder, and there can be increased heat emission over the affected bones due to the increased amount of blood flow.

If no symptoms are reported by the patient, then treatment is not required. However, in patients complaining of pain, a hormone (calcitonin) injected subcutaneously is often effective. A nasal spray is now available as well. Bisphosphonates (chemicals that restrict bone destruction) can also help. They are available in oral form; however, this medication is usually not used more than six months because of changes in bone mineralization.

Infectious Arthritis

Infectious arthritis is an infection of the joint by bacteria inside the joint, and it causes an intense, painful inflammatory process. The illness is seen in people who have previously damaged a joint. It is also seen in intravenous drug abusers. Nongonococcal acute bacterial arthritis (septic arthritis), a type of infectious arthritis, is a very serious medical emergency requiring removal of infected joint fluid daily and intravenous antibiotics.

The most common bacterial cause of infectious arthritis is *Staphylococcus aureus*. Usually there is an additional infection outside the joint, and the patient may be acutely ill. Occasionally this type of acute infection follows arthroscopy (a surgical procedure in which the surface of the bones are viewed by a surgeon). The infection may also occur with joint replacement surgery. This is a very serious condition and can be fatal, particularly in neglected cases.

Gonococcal arthritis is another acute infectious arthritic syndrome, and it is the most common cause of infectious arthritis in urban areas. This illness can occur in otherwise healthy individuals, unlike the other forms of infectious arthritis described above. Many people don't know that it is possible to have gonorrhea with no symptoms and that it may involve tissues outside the genitals, including the throat and rectal area.

Approximately 50 percent of those afflicted with this disorder also have a severe infection in one joint. Prior to this, they may have experienced pain in other joints, which could be fleeting in nature.

Patients with this disorder should be hospitalized and started on intravenous antibiotics. The reason for hospitalization is that in recent years, the gonococcus (the bacterium causing the disorder) is resistant to many different types of antibiotics. Individuals suffering from the human immunodeficiency virus (HIV) also often have arthritic complaints. They may have Reiter's syndrome or other types of arthritis. It is not clear if these arthritic problems are a direct consequence of the HIV infection or are from other infections that can occur in people who are HIV positive.

Viral syndromes can also affect joints. Mumps, hepatitis, and other viruses can lead to an arthritis associated with the infection. There is usually no specific therapy for such arthritis; rather, when the infection resolves, the arthritis resolves.

Fibromyalgia (Fibrositis)

Fibromyalgia is a fairly widespread disorder; symptoms include diffuse pain in the musculoskeletal system as well as stiffness, lack of stamina, and difficulty achieving restful sleep. Occasionally numbness and tingling symptoms can be present, predominantly in women between the ages of twenty-five and forty-five.

The cause of fibromyalgia is unknown but may be related to a disturbance in certain segments of the normal sleep cycle. One study performed on normal subjects who were awakened as soon as they achieved a sleep stage revealed symptoms very similar to this disorder. Stress, unrelated medical illness, thyroid disease, and trauma have often been mentioned as causative mechanisms in fibromyalgia. It has been described in HIV infection as well and in Lyme disease.

People afflicted with fibromyalgia are tired most of the time and are very stiff, usually in the morning, although most people improve during the day. Cold or damp weather, anxiety, and stress can make the patient's symptoms worse. Over-exertion can also exacerbate the condition. Migraine, irritable bowel syndrome, and disturbances in the menstruation cycle are often encountered in individuals with this diagnosis.

Patients have specific, very tender areas upon local pressure. Often these tender sites (trigger points) radiate to other areas nearby. The tender spots are in the supporting musculature of the neck and at many other sites, particularly at the shoulder girdle. This is usually not a serious condition in terms of significant disability. Heat, massage, and even injection of the tender sites with local anesthetics can be helpful, as can an intelligent exercise program. Sleep habits should also be examined.

Lyme Disease (Lyme Borreliosis)

This is an infectious disease caused by a spirochete (form of bacteria similar to syphilis) that is transmitted to humans through ticks. The disease typically follows a course with three fairly well-delineated stages.

In the first stage, the patient develops flu-like symptoms and a characteristic rash (erythema migrans). The flu-like symptom is seen in about half the patients and usually involves diffuse muscle pain and even chills and fever. The rash usually appears about a week after the tick bite but may not appear for a full month. A flat or possibly slightly raised red lesion appears at the site of the tick bite. Over several days, this lesion begins to disappear from the center outward. About 20 percent of the people who develop Lyme disease don't notice the lesion. These symptoms resolve within a month.

The second stage marks the traveling of the spirochete via the blood or lymph system to other organs, usually a few weeks later. Symptoms may occur in the skin, nervous system, and the musculoskeletal system. Often headache and neck stiffness are symptoms, as well as pain in the tendons, muscles, and joints. Extreme fatigue and a general sense of being ill (malaise) often occur. Serious cardiac disease may occur during this stage, and some patients suffer nerve injuries or meningitis and even occasionally develop a brain infection (encephalitis).

The third stage may occur on a very delayed basis, up to years after the infection. Up to 60 percent of those with Lyme disease will later develop musculoskeletal problems. These symptoms can be quite variable in nature and may involve severe joint pain and pain in the areas surrounding the joints as well as a severe arthritis of large joints.

A chronic inflammation of the synovial membrane can be quite severe and may lead to destruction of joints and significant disability. The cause for these delayed musculoskeletal joint injuries is unclear but is thought to be related to some type of immunologic cause. Antibiotics are often effective in treating many symptoms but often not the arthritic problems.

A situation will arise in which patients have joint pain and a positive blood test for Lyme disease, which is notoriously unreliable. These patients will often request antibiotic therapy, which can cost up to $5,000. It should be remembered that Lyme disease is primarily a clinical diagnosis, and there is no test that is completely reliable for this disorder.

Overuse Syndromes (Repetitive Strain Injuries)

Some injuries appear to be associated with repetitive use of particular parts of the body. This can lead to nerve entrapments such as carpal tunnel syndrome, small fractures in bones, often of the feet, as well as tendinitis and bursitis. Muscle pain is very often a consequence of this type of injury.

When the muscle is involved, it appears that the use of the muscle exceeds the muscle's ability to repair itself, which leads to actual destruction and pain in the muscle involved. These types of injuries are common causes of arm and leg discomfort.

Therapy typically consists of resting the affected area, combined with various types of treatments, including massage. We discuss various types of treatment for arthritis pain in Chapter 7.

Myofascial Pain Syndrome

Myofascial pain syndrome is not a term describing a pain in your face. Instead, it refers to chronic pain related to a muscle and its covering (fascia). It usually occurs in response to an injury in which muscle fibers are actually torn, such as a whiplash injury.

Pain continues because of muscle spasms and knots, which are trigger points in the muscles. This can be a very difficult injury to treat, although it does often respond to chiropractic care, physical therapy, massage, and medications. Frequently, injections of a local anesthetic into these trigger points are effective. Stretching and strengthening exercises are often helpful in reducing the muscle pain that comes with this syndrome.

Nerve Entrapment Syndromes

Pinched nerves in the hand (carpal tunnel syndrome) can lead to wrist and hand pain that might be confused with osteoarthritis. Nerve entrapment syndrome is associated with weakness and numbness of the hand. Symptoms are most severe at night and can awaken the person from a sound sleep.

A similar syndrome, tarsal syndrome, is related to a pinched nerve near the ankle. Symptoms of this problem include radiating pain into the thigh or into the foot. This illness is often confused with foot and ankle arthritic disease.

Pinched nerves in the neck frequently radiate into the shoulder and can cause confusion in diagnosis. It is quite common for individuals with pinched nerves in the neck to develop shoulder pain as well and to experience the diminished use of the affected shoulder. This in turn can lead to intense shoulder pain and loss of range of motion (frozen shoulder syndrome). Frozen shoulder syndrome usually responds to the manipulation of the shoulder through normal range of motion while the patient is under complete anesthesia.

Pain whose source is the lower joints of the spine (facet joints) can appear as pain in the hip. The phenomenon of pain appearing in a place different from its source is called referred pain. People who complain to their doctors of hip pain may actually have a back problem. The facet syndrome (inflammation in the facet joint) frequently responds to exercise, muscle strengthening, activity modification, and local injection.

Restless Leg Syndrome

Restless leg syndrome (RLS) is a condition that may affect up to 15 percent of the population. Like osteoarthritis, it is a common disorder and should be considered in individuals complaining of leg discomfort. Patients with nerve disease (polyneuropathy) are often thought to have restless leg syndrome when they actually have cramping related to the nerve disease.

RLS can appear at any age, but almost half the patients report some symptoms before the age of twenty. Approximately two-thirds of the patients who describe symptoms consistent with restless leg syndrome report that it worsens with age. Usually RLS affects both legs. Individuals with this disorder complain of an unpleasant sensation in their legs. It may not be reported as pain, although many patients say they experience a deep, severe aching discomfort in both legs. Patients often report a creeping sensation and a crawling numbness, as well as a burning or tingling in the area. They gain some relief by moving about. The sensations are worse in the late evening and night, and people affected with RLS feel compelled to move their legs.

Patients have great difficulty getting a restful sleep at night and often have repetitive movements of the legs while asleep (these can be discovered in a routine sleep evaluation). Restless leg syndrome can be seen in a number of conditions, including vitamin B_{12} deficiency, kidney failure, Parkinson's disease, pregnancy, and pinched nerves in the low back.

Treatment for RLS includes correcting the underlying problem if found; also, a variety of medications are available, and you should ask your physician which one might be right for you. Neurologists and sleep specialists have a great deal of experience dealing with this disorder.

Now that we've gone through the maze of possible illnesses that may mimic arthritis, we'll talk about how you and your doctor, together, can come to the correct diagnosis and what you can do about it!

3

Your Visit with the Doctor

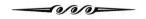

L et's say you don't have a doctor. Maybe you're new in town, or your doctor has retired and you've forgotten who your records have been sent to. You're having a flare-up of what could be arthritis, and you are in major pain!

When you're in the throes of an arthritic attack, you may be very tempted to open up the phone book and find a name that has an M.D. after it in the "Physicians" listing. Resist this impulse! Instead, take some over-the-counter painkillers; when you've recovered enough to use your usual good judgment, follow the guidelines provided here. (If the pain is very severe, go to the hospital emergency room.)

In this chapter, we'll talk about how to find a good doctor, how to evaluate your new (or "old,"—if you have one now) doctor, and how to create and maintain a good relationship once you do find a physician you feel you can work with. These guidelines are important because they can steer you directly to good care, which in turn leads to less pain for you. We offer some clear do's and don'ts to follow.

Also, in this chapter we'll talk about the physical examination: how to prepare for it so you don't waste your precious time and what happens during the typical visit. In addition, we'll talk about tests that your doctor may order. Some of these tests are specifically oriented to the person who may have osteoarthritis, while others are used to diagnose an array of disorders.

Choosing the Right Doctor

Okay, so you've resisted the urge to open the phone book to the doctors section, close your eyes, and stab your finger at one of the names at random. So what's the right way to find yourself a good physician?

- If you already have a family practitioner or internist, ask who he or she would recommend. Keep in mind that the doctor may wish to diagnose and treat you first and then, if unable to resolve your problem, refer you to a specialist. This is especially true if you are under a managed care system. (More on managed care later in this chapter.) It's a good idea to ask a doctor you already know and trust to recommend an expert in pain management, because good doctors work with other good doctors. In fact, your doctor's staff may even set up the appointment for you, probably getting you in much earlier than if you tried to make the appointment by yourself.

- If you don't have a regular doctor or your physician doesn't recommend someone, you could discuss the problem with friends who have osteoarthritis and pain. They may have located a doctor who is an expert in pain management. Keep in mind, however, that people are different—just because your friend likes a doctor does not mean you will like that person too.

- Check with your reference librarian at the public library to see if any physicians in your local area have published articles or books on acute or chronic pain, joint pain, or arthritis. You may even wish to review what the doctor has written (if it is not in a complicated medical journal full of jargon), so you can get an idea of what this doctor thinks and believes.

- If you are in serious pain and over-the-counter painkillers just don't give you any adequate relief, one fallback position is the hospital emergency room (ER). Doctors in the ER treat people who walk in with a broad variety of complaints, and they should be able to recommend a physician who can treat you as an outpatient later on. One caution: The hospital will usually recommend you only to doctors on its staff, and Doctor Perfect might be on staff at another hospital in your area.

A Look at Managed Care

Managed care has permeated much of society today, and consequently some people believe they have lost control over who they may see. They say, "I don't have any choice. I must see a physician on my plan." While we have no control in choosing our parents or our brothers and sisters—we can't even really control how our own children will turn out—we can absolutely choose our spouses and friends, and often we can choose our physicians as well.

If you do find a doctor who you feel can alleviate your pain but for whatever reason is not on your HMO, PPO, or other managed care list, don't give up right away. Insurance companies often have an option for an out-of-network provider—in other words, a doctor who's not on their list. You usually pay one rate or some percentage of a fee for the in-network doctors (the ones on the list) and a slightly higher rate for the out-of-network doctors.

Find out if your insurance company does have a provision for out-of-network coverage. Call your insurance company or talk to your insurance representative at work, and be sure to talk to a supervisor (the first response you'll get from some clerks is "No," because they don't want to bother looking for the correct answer). Write down what you're told by the managed care rep—it's easy to get confused.

If your insurance company does have out-of-network coverage, the next step is to ask the insurance company if you need to write a letter before the doctor visit or if the doctor (or you) can submit a claim after the visit. If so, try to find a reason for the visit that sounds like it would save money, over the long or short haul, because that's what motivates many insurance companies these days. How bad or sad you feel probably won't move the person who reads your letter, but if there's a chance some dollars could be saved—that gets attention.

Even if your insurance company has no provision for out-of-network coverage, you may still wish to see a doctor who is not on its managed care list, if you think that person can resolve your pain better than anyone else. To save some money, perhaps the new, out-of-network doctor would be willing to have your in-network physician order any lab work or special tests and then forward them; that way, you'd be responsible for the doctor's fee only. Be sure to talk to the new doctor about this before you make arrangements. After the out-of-network doctor diagnoses you and begins treatment, he or she may be able to turn your case back to the in-network doctor, perhaps following up once a year or as needed. Also, often we will see patients for an evaluation and summary assessment, to provide a clear diagnosis and to outline a short- and long-term treatment plan.

Questions to Ask the Doctor

Okay, you're in the treatment room and you're ready to see the doctor. Do you just sit there and passively follow orders and respond to questions? No! You do not. Seek an interactive, collaborative relationship, in which both you and the doctor participate. The list that follows are some questions you may wish to ask the doctor.

- Ask the doctor if arthritis is a particular interest. Some doctors think arthritis is boring, or they may not treat many patients with arthritis and thus do not keep up with the latest research on treatments and medications. Most doctors are adept at treating illnesses with which they have experience.
- Some doctors refuse to prescribe pain medications. This is another problem area to watch out for. Ask the doctor how he or she treats pain. If the very first response is, "I won't give you medicines for pain," you should see this as a red flag and a very bad sign. While a doctor should not rely on pain medication only, refusing to even consider medicine is an indicator that this may not be the doctor for you.
- Ask if the doctor uses a variety of different medications or relies mostly on one or two. The doctor may volunteer this information when you ask about medications, but to be clear, ask again: "Doctor Kildare, are you saying that you rely mostly on *abc* and *xyz* for chronic pain?" "Doctor Welby, do you mean that there are many different medicines that might work?" The doctor will agree with you if you've understood the information and correct you if you haven't. If the doctor relies heavily on one or two medications, consider this as another red flag. Many medications are available to treat arthritis, and new ones are being developed all the time. The tried-and-true medication might be just right for you—or it might not be.

Other Questions to Ask

In addition to actually talking to the doctor, there are a variety of good ways to evaluate if a doctor is the right person for you. Following are three items to consider:

- Timewise, are you and the doctor pretty much in synch with each other? For example, if you are a clock-watcher who can't stand lateness and the doctor consistently runs thirty or more minutes late, then you two probably aren't a good match; or, if you're fairly relaxed about time and you get to your appointment within ten minutes but your doctor has everything very tightly scheduled, then that probably won't work, either. If you're not a good fit for each other, then you should continue your search, whenever possible.

- What is the doctor's staff like? If the first words out of the staff person's mouth are, "And how will you be paying for this—cash, check, or credit card?" then this is a bad sign. The staff should greet you politely. A new patient will need to give payment information, but that should not be the only thing that the staff seems to care about.

- Does the doctor care about advance preparation? One way to know is if the staff asks you about recent medical records the doctor could look at. This indicates they are interested in helping you resolve your medical problem. It's also a good sign that the doctor wants to be as well prepared as possible even before you walk through the door.

Your Examination

Whenever you can, it's a good idea to be prepared ahead of time before your visit to your doctor, whether it's your first visit or fifty-first visit. Knowing what to bring with you to the examination and having an idea of what to expect during it can remove much of the mystery and anxiety of an impending doctor visit—especially if this is your first encounter with the doctor. If the initial visit goes well, it often sets a solid foundation for an effective doctor-patient relationship that can last for years.

When you go to your exam, have the following items with you:

- Previous medical records
- Prior diagnostic testing, x-rays, and lab reports
- A list of other treating physicians, especially those who are out of state or out of the general area. Whether local or not, include their phone numbers (or, even better, their business cards).

In order to have enough time to amass the information just described, be sure that you call ahead to doctors' offices, x-ray departments, and so forth at least two to three weeks before the date of your appointment. Pick them up about two days before the visit with your new doctor and not on the same day (you don't need any additional stress!).

Some doctors' offices refuse to release medical records directly to patients; instead, they insist on sending records directly to the new doctor. Unfortunately, sending out records is often such a low priority that the staff may forget about it altogether. So to avoid this problem, if the office refuses to give you your records, ask when the records will be mailed. Then call the new doctor's office four or five days after that date to verify that the records have actually arrived. If they have not, call the sending office and ask the staff to please check that the records were sent, because the new doctor really needs the important information compiled by the previous doctor's extremely efficient staff.

Your Medical History

The main information exchange from you to the doctor occurs when you answer the doctor's questions about your medical history. Often, 80 percent of any diagnosis is made up of the clinical information that the doctor elicits from you, and the more accurate the data, the better. Computer lovers call it "garbage in, garbage out," which means if you provide bad data, you get bad results.

Many doctors who treat arthritis will give you a pain questionnaire before the visit, but don't be surprised if the doctor asks you the same or similar questions in person. There is a reason for this: many times, a patient may forget something while in the waiting room filling out a questionnaire, but the memory is jogged when the doctor asks the same question face to face.

Questions Your Doctor May Ask

As with any illness, your doctor will ask when your symptoms occur, how frequent they are, how long they last (minutes, hours, days), and if you get any relief. Rating the severity of your pain is important too, because your physician needs to be able to determine if you are getting better or worse or staying about the same. The doctor will also be looking for patterns of symptoms and activities that seem to be related to (or may cause) the symptoms. Your doctor will also ask about any therapies or actions that seem to alleviate the symptoms. Be prepared with answers to the questions that follow.

What medications are you now taking? Every good doctor wants to know what medicines you are on now. It's also a good idea to tell your doctor about medications you have tried in the past for similar symptoms. Tell the doctor if they helped you at all and also report on any side effects or problems that you experienced while taking them.

We recommend that you "clean out your medicine chest," and by that we mean pull out all the medicines you regularly or frequently take and put them in an oversized, clear plastic bag for your doctor's visit. Don't forget over-the-counter drugs that you are taking very often—sometimes these medications can contribute to your problem. And bring in any "natural" treatments, too—if you're taking them to try to help your problem, show them to your doctor.

Do external factors seem to affect you? Your doctor should be very interested in outside factors that may trigger your symptoms, whether changes in the weather or barometric pressure, stress, hormonal changes, or others. What about your sleep habits? If you sleep well, does anything change? If you are having trouble sleeping, does the pain level change? Your doctor may also ask about sexual activity, which is a reasonable topic to pursue. Do you get better or worse if you smoke or drink alcohol or use caffeine? All of this information is important and will help your doctor help you. Do not withhold information because you're afraid the doctor will lecture you for smoking, drinking, and so on. If you are using other substances, for example, marijuana, be sure to include that fact in your discussion. Your doctor needs good information to come to the right diagnosis.

What is your emotional state? Your overall mind-set, energy level, and stamina are important factors to your doctor, as well as any irritability, moodiness, or bad temper. We'll talk much more about this issue in Chapter 11.

What is your family medical history? Your doctor will also usually ask you about other people in your family who may have the same medical problems. Many illnesses have a genetic component. So if your mother and father have arthritis, you may have inherited a predisposition. If you were adopted or for some reason do not have this information, don't worry, your doctor will still be able to treat you.

The Physical Examination

After taking your complete medical history, the doctor will begin the physical examination of your body. While some physicians take out a stethoscope and listen to the heart and lungs, calling that a "complete" exam, we don't agree. Instead, we prefer to examine our patients in a partially undressed state, wearing a hospital gown that we provide. The hospital gown allows the doctor to see muscles, limbs, and joints, as well as the entire spine, a major source for arthritic pain.

After a general assessment, the pain specialist will examine and evaluate your joints, including the cervical, thoracic, and lumbar spine, the hips and pelvis, and the major and minor joints. The doctor will be checking for your range of motion (how much and how far you can move your joints), joint swelling, and "angry joints," which seem hot or inflamed. The doctor will often evaluate your overall mood, judgment, and speed of thought, to determine your ability to concentrate.

Testing your motor strength, how you walk and stand, and your balance are all part of a neurologic exam. The neurologic exam is the formal testing of the brain, the spinal cord, the nerve roots that come out of the spinal cord, and the muscles that these nerve roots send messages to. Don't be surprised if the doctor asks you to walk on your heels or toes up and down the hallway. These observations can tell the doctor a lot, not only about your spine but also about your joints and the weight-bearing aspects of your muscles and skeletal system.

The Next Step

After the history and the physical exam are both completed, what happens next depends on a variety of factors. If your condition is a chronic one and it has been well documented through diagnostic testing, laboratory testing, and so on, then the next step may be a therapeutic intervention. Often, no additional tests will be needed; however, in many cases of chronic arthritis or an acute attack of arthritis pain, the doctor may obtain additional tests, such as special imaging studies or laboratory tests (especially blood tests).

X-Rays

Doctors have been using x-rays for more than a century, but the equipment and techniques used today are completely different and far more effective. In fact, processes have changed radically in the past ten years alone. X-rays also can be extremely useful in detecting many spinal and joint disorders. When performed in context with a thorough physical examination and an accurate medical history, the x-ray is often the only test needed to enable the doctor to diagnose you.

An x-ray technician may take x-rays of anterior and posterior views (front to back), the lateral view (side), and/or oblique (diagonal). Sometimes certain joints are also x-rayed. Often, simple x-rays can reveal wear and tear changes on the joints and the discs, as well as show evidence of swelling and fractures. Unfortunately, it is easy to miss a hairline fracture with a simple x-ray.

Still, as a general rule, structural and weight-bearing areas of the body can be accurately assessed with x-rays. Bone spurs, or wear and tear changes on the bones (which look like the pointy parts of sea coral), can be seen readily with x-rays. In fact, these bone spurs can be missed with the more expensive and complicated MRI test. The x-ray is also a good study for the joints of the spine. Spondylolisthesis, a condition in which the vertebrae of the spine have separated from the bony arches, can be visualized well with simple x-rays.

X-rays can also often identify serious conditions, such as bone cancer and osteoporosis (bone loss), as well as numerous other conditions. It's a quick, useful, and relatively inexpensive diagnostic test.

The disadvantage of x-rays is that they do not show the soft tissues of the body. With just an x-ray, often a doctor must guess at a problem of the soft tissue, ligament, or tendon as well as a problem with the intervertebral discs (the shock absorbers between the bones of the spine).

Magnetic Resonance Imaging (MRI)

The MRI is an exciting and relatively recent technique many doctors use to diagnose a variety of medical problems. This test works through magnetic fields that alter the orientation of molecules in the body's tissues. It's completely safe.

The MRI can help in revealing problems not only in the neck, mid back, and low back but also in multiple joints of the body. It is also effective in showing the knee, hip, shoulder, and wrist joints, as well as your finger and toe joints.

The MRI should not be used alone, with no x-rays; instead it should be a complementary study. Together, the x-ray and the MRI can provide your doctor with a look at both the hard and soft tissue of a joint or structure causing you pain.

An MRI is expensive and costs over a thousand dollars. Another problem with the MRI is that some patients object to the tightly confined spaces in which the MRI must be done for an optimum scan of the body. Patients who are claustrophobic should tell their doctor ahead of time—a mild tranquilizer taken before the test might help. (Of course, if you take a tranquilizer before leaving home, you should have someone drive you to the doctor's office and back home again.)

You can't have an MRI if you have some types of artificial heart valves, a pacemaker, or metal clips placed in your body during prior surgery. If the doctor schedules an MRI and does not ask you about these circumstances, speak up!

Bone Scans

Doctors have been using bone scans for decades. Inflammation, infection, and cancer typically cause an increased concentration of radioactive isotope. The patient is given an initial injection of a radioactive isotope and asked to come back a few hours later. Usually, a series of images are taken. The radioactive isotope collects in greater amounts where there are areas of abnormal bone. A bone scan can be performed on specific sections as well as the entire skeletal system, thus making it a very useful screening technique.

The bone scan exposes you to a minimal amount of radiation. Another negative aspect is that the procedure requires you to lie flat on your back for some period of time, which could be very uncomfortable if you're having joint and spine pain.

Bone Density Studies

Bone density studies screen the density of the mineralization of your bones and are very effective at detecting osteoporosis. If you do have osteoporosis, treatments often include hormone therapy, exercise, and resistance training and some medications.

This study is usually fairly comfortable and is not invasive. Doctors can also compare the results of your bone study to people who are the same age and sex. The doctor may also use the study as a baseline, ordering a new one several years later to see if there have been any changes.

Physical Capacity Evaluation/ Physical Therapy Assessment

Often at the onset of a treatment plan, doctors also order a general physical therapy evaluation, to help them determine any restriction of your range of motion or any instability of the joints, pelvic tilt, spinal curvature, and so forth. (See Chapter 7 for more information on physical therapy.)

Creating and Maintaining a Good Doctor-Patient Relationship

You've found a good doctor who has diagnosed and treated your problem, and you're satisfied with him or her. Don't assume there's nothing more for you to do, because the fact is that a variety of important factors affect the success of your relationship with your physician. Some of these are your own honest attitude, your willingness to communicate, and your resistance of the common tendency to self-diagnose! Also, remember that your doctor is a person, not a superhero.

Be Honest with Yourself and the Doctor

In developing a good relationship with your new (or current) doctors, it's important to recognize what you are and are not willing to do (or can't do). For example, if the doctor believes that stress is a major problem for you, and you believe that the cause of the stress (your marriage, your kids, your job) cannot be changed, then be frank and say so.

In addition, if the physician wants you to give up smoking, lose fifty pounds, or take some other action, and you know you are not willing or can't do it, tell your doctor. Perhaps you could cut back on smoking or lose ten pounds. Or maybe you aren't willing to go that far—which is a bad idea, but it's better to be up front about it. It makes no sense for a physician to outline a treatment plan that you won't comply with.

Doctors Are Human!

We want you to always remember that your doctor is a mortal being. Some people (and some doctors!) think that physicians are gods. Most doctors are very smart and very caring people, but that does not mean they know all and see all. If your doctor doesn't know everything about a new drug or treatment you've just seen on the six o'clock news, that doesn't mean your doctor is not competent.

Good doctors keep up on the latest medical research, usually through their medical journals. Sometimes patients read about just-breaking stories in popular magazines (or hear it on the news); these stories haven't made it to the medical journals yet, which can lead to problems. For example, news of a major breakthrough on migraine headaches first "broke" in *People* magazine. The very next day after the article appeared, our office was flooded with phone calls regarding the "miracle medicine." Unfortunately, the article in *People* didn't talk about the general indications for the use of the medicine, restrictions on its use, side effects, and so forth. Callers were demanding this new drug, when often it wasn't right for them at all!

Popular shows, such as *60 Minutes*, sometimes have "investigative reports" that may lead you to believe there are serious problems with a medication or treatment. Instead of calling up your doctor in a panic and saying, "Doctor, I think this medicine will kill me! I know, because I saw it on *60 Minutes!*"—take a different approach. Tell your doctor you're worried about something you've just heard and ask if there's any substance or validity to it. The doctor may explain that the show was sensationalistic and there is no problem with a medication or treatment. Or, there may be problems or side effects associated with the medication, but you would be much worse without the drug. Your doctor can explain the pros and cons to you and is far more likely to give you the information you need. Physicians are sworn to "do no harm." Let them adhere to that credo!

Of course, it's perfectly reasonable and a good idea to ask the doctor why a certain drug, treatment, or regimen is recommended. If you don't understand what you're supposed to do and why you are supposed to do it, it will affect your motivation and overall compliance with what the doctor ordered.

Cooperation with Your Doctor Is Important

Maintain a positive mental attitude! This is hard to do when you don't feel well, but it is well worth the effort. Remember that the doctor's goal is to empower you to take charge of your own health. Getting you to a higher level of wellness may take some time, but remember that the responsibility for a satisfactory outcome must be *shared*. We perform many free public seminars on a variety of topics, including arthritis, spine pain, and migraines. One of the themes that we stress is open communication. To make our point, we show a slide of a golfer in a sand trap asking his caddie for a sand wedge. Instead of a sand wedge, he is handed a sandwich. If you are asking your doctor for one thing, and your doctor isn't hearing you or is providing you with something else, that's a problem.

Consider yourself a person who provides clues to your doctor, who is your medical Sherlock Holmes, zeroing in on what the problem really is and the consequent best solution to solve it.

Don't Self-Diagnose

One *very* important point is that you should not be too hasty about self-diagnosis. Tell the doctor about past diagnoses and answer questions, but allow the doctor to make his or her own judgment calls. Rather than say, "I'm here to get treatment for my osteoarthritis," it's better to tell the doctor about your list of symptoms, complaints, and processes. As a result of your self-diagnosis, if your doctor doesn't identify a serious treatable condition (one that you may not know about), it could lead to serious complications for you.

This point was brought home to us recently. Another physician was treating a patient we'll call "Don" for spine pain. Don had suddenly stopped taking his medicine because he said he did not want to "live with pain pills." He was soon thereafter seen in the hospital emergency room, complaining of abdominal pain. Don told doctors there that it was "probably medication withdrawal" making him sick, and they accepted this explanation.

A cursory examination didn't reveal anything significant, and Don was hospitalized and monitored for withdrawal symptoms. But he got worse—Don's pain level increased markedly. We were consulted because of the escalating pain. By the time we saw Don, his blood count had plummeted and he had developed a hemorrhage in his abdomen. We promptly diagnosed him, and Don was taken to the operating room for a ruptured spleen, which was removed.

Don has healed well and is now back to jogging three to four miles per day. But he was a very sick man until properly diagnosed.

The doctor listened to Don's self-diagnosis of being "in withdrawal." Without learning additional information—such as the fact that Don recently had a trauma to his abdominal wall and had developed a bruise there—the ER doctor could not possibly have diagnosed him properly. Don't make the mistake that Don made. Do not fall into the self-diagnosis trap.

Conclusion

When diagnosing problems related to arthritis, whether the problem occurs in the joints of the spine or major or minor joints of other parts of the musculoskeletal system, the modern doctor has very sophisticated tools available. Ultimately, however, a smart doctor relies heaviest on the patient's medical history and a careful physical examination, which provide the most reliable and cost-effective sources of information.

Many physicians treat arthritis pain: neurologists (like us), physiatrists, rheumatologists, internists, family practitioners, gynecologists, and chiropractic physicians. Indeed, chiropractors are often at their best when it comes to arthritis disorders of the spine. What's more important than the type of doctor is whether the doctor is interested in the disorder and is skilled at diagnosis and management of both acute and chronic arthritis pain.

Once your doctor launches you on a treatment plan, the goal is for you to have greatly diminished pain—perhaps even a pain-free existence—and a happier and more productive life.

4

Traditional Drug Therapy

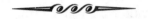

Nearly everyone who suffers from arthritis has taken a medication of some sort to propel them through the pain, and you may well be one of them. Perhaps you've taken an over-the-counter pain medication or a medicine that your doctor prescribed, or both.

Most medications are prescribed on a temporary basis, although some medications must be taken every day for years or even a lifetime. In our practice, we frequently prescribe medications for our patients with arthritic complaints, particularly spinal arthritis. We recognize that a person who is in constant pain will usually not recover as quickly as a person who is pain-free or who has a low level of pain. However, we prefer that our patients take medication only to alleviate the pain. Our goal is to get the patient to a comfortable level, initiate the appropriate therapy, then have our patient taper off the medication for good.

A key reason for our policy is that all medications can have side effects, and some can be quite serious. For example, acetaminophen—which you may know by its most common brand name, Tylenol—can have serious side effects if used on a prolonged basis or incorrectly.

In this chapter, we discuss medications for arthritis, particularly classes of medications used for pain management. We'll discuss the various side effects and the expected positive benefits from the various medications. We'll explain why doctors sometimes switch from medication to medication and why some medications are used in combinations.

Most medications can be administered through various methods, including by mouth, by injection, by nasal spray, and by skin patch. Medications can also be given by rectal suppository. The method your doctor chooses will depend on the type of medication as well as the frequency and the dosage required.

Remember, the timing of your medication usage is important. If you wait until the pain is severe, then you will often need a larger dose of pain medication to "catch up" to the pain and obtain adequate relief. Think of medications as soldiers fighting on your behalf. Send your "troops" into battle early on, and you'll have a far better chance of affecting a positive outcome. On the other hand, dosing too many times could lead to toxicity and possibly addiction.

When pain becomes severe and joints don't work and muscles or ligaments can't move, often the only recourse is to visit the emergency room, which can be a nightmarish affair. Emergency room doctors are trained to take care of critically ill patients with strokes, heart attacks, gunshot wounds, and other major trauma; as a result, they can be insensitive to the exquisite agony of acute joint pain syndrome, thinking, hey, it's "just" arthritis.

For example, Jill, a patient we've followed for some time for her multiple joint and muscle pains, at one time slipped and fell, suffering an acute flare-up. As anyone who has experienced arthritis pain can attest, acute pain on top of chronic pain can be unbearable. To make things worse, the fall occurred on a Saturday afternoon. She went to the local ER, checked in, and waited. And waited. And waited. Meanwhile, Jill's pain became much worse. By the time she was seen, she couldn't stand or walk—her knee joints and hip joints were so inflamed, they just couldn't work. Jill ultimately had to be admitted to the hospital for pain management and physical therapy. Take your medication as soon as symptoms start to flare up, and avoid emergency room visits.

Commonly Used Medications

In this section, we will discuss medications that are frequently used to alleviate joint pain, including over-the-counter and prescribed medicines. Some of them will be familiar names, and others may be new to you.

Nonsteroidal Anti-Inflammatory Drugs (NSAIDs)

Anti-inflammatories are traditionally quite useful for controlling pain, swelling, and inflammation. They are also effective in reducing joint inflammation. NSAIDs are generally safe, but they should be used with caution. They can be particularly harmful to individuals with gastrointestinal (stomach) or renal (kidney) problems. Many of them are available without a prescription.

There are six chemical classes of anti-inflammatories; they are summarized in Table 4.1. Your doctor not only can choose from within one class of medicine but also can switch from class to class of anti-inflammatory agent. You'll find descriptions of the six classes in the following sections.

Salicylic Acids   Aspirin is the most commonly recognized form of salicylic acid and was probably the first NSAID developed. It is very effective for most benign types of arthritic pain and is also very effective for mild to moderate pain. According to some estimates, at least 20,000 tons of aspirin are consumed in this country each year—that's forty million pounds!

Table 4.1 NONSTEROIDAL ANTI-INFLAMMATORY DRUGS
CLASS, DOSAGE STRENGTHS, AND INDICATIONS

Drug Class	Dosage Strengths and Forms	OA*	RA*	Pain
Pyranocarboxylic Acids				
Lodine® (etodolac)	200 mg 300 mg 400 mg 500 mg	✔	✔	✔
Arylacetic Acids				
Cataflam® (diclofenae potassium)	200 mg	✔	✔	✔
Clinoril® (sulindac)	150 mg 200 mg	✔	✔	
Indocin® (indomethacin)	25 mg 50 mg	✔	✔	
Indocin® SR (indomethacin)	75 mg	✔	✔	
Tolectin® (tolmetin sodium)	200 mg 400 mg 600 mg	✔	✔	
Toradol® (ketorolac tromethamine)	10 mg			✔
Voltaren® (diclofenac sodium)	25 mg 50 mg 75 mg	✔	✔	
Voltaren® XR (diclofenac sodium)	100 mg	✔	✔	
Propionic Acids				
Anaprox® (naproxen sodium)	275 mg	✔	✔	✔
Anaprox® DS (naproxen sodium)	550 mg	✔	✔	✔
Ansaid® (flurbiprofen)	50 mg 100 mg	✔	✔	
Daypro® (oxaprozin)	600 mg	✔	✔	
EC-Naprosyn® (naproxen)	375 mg 500 mg	✔	✔	
Motrin® (ibuprofen)	300 mg 400 mg 600 mg 800 mg	✔	✔	✔
Naprelan® (naproxen sodium)	375 mg 500 mg	✔	✔	✔
Naprosyn® (naproxen)	250 mg 375 mg 500 mg	✔	✔	✔
Naprosyn® suspension (naproxen)	125 mg/5 mL	✔	✔	✔
Orudis® (ketoprofen)	25 mg 50 mg 75 mg	✔	✔	✔
Oruvail® (ketoprofen)	100 mg 150 mg 200 mg	✔	✔	
Salicylic Acids				
aspirin		✔	✔	✔
Disalcid™ (salsalate)	500 mg 500 mg 750 mg	✔	✔	

Table 4.1 NONSTEROIDAL ANTI-INFLAMMATORY DRUGS
CLASS, DOSAGE STRENGTHS, AND INDICATIONS *(continued)*

Drug Class	Dosage Strengths and Forms	Indications OA*	RA*	Pain
Dolobid® (diflunisal)	250 mg 500 mg	✔	✔	
Mono-Gesic® (salsalate)	750 mg	✔	✔	
Salflex® (salsalate)	500 mg 750 mg	✔	✔	
Oxicans				
Feldene® (piroxicam)	10 mg 20 mg	✔	✔	
Naphthylalkanones				
Relafen® (nabumetone)	500 mg 750 mg	✔	✔	

*OA = Osteoarthritis; RA = Rheumatoid Arthritis

The most frequent complaints with NSAIDs relate to the GI tract. Serious GI toxicity such as perforation, ulceration, and bleeding can occur in patients treated chronically with NSAID therapy.

Lodine, Naprelan, Orudis, and Oruvail are registered trademarks of Wyeth-Ayerst Laboratories; Cataflam and Voltaren are registered trademarks of Geigy Pharmaceuticals; Clinoril, Indocin, and Dolobid are registered trademarks of Merck & Co., Inc.; Tolectin is a registered trademark of McNeil Pharmaceutical; Anaprox and Toradol are registered trademarks of Roche Laboratories; Naprosyn is a registered trademark and EC-Naprosyn is a trademark of Syntex Puerto Rico, Inc.; Ansaid and Motrin are registered trademarks of The Upjohn Company; Daypro is a registered trademark of G.D. Searle & Co.; Disalcid is a trademark of 3M Pharmaceuticals; Mono-Gesic is a registered trademark of Central Pharmaceuticals, Inc.; Salflex is a registered trademark of Camrick Laboratories, Inc.; Feldene is a registered trademark of Pratt Pharmaceuticals; Relafen is a registered trademark of SmithKline Beecham Pharmaceuticals.

Aspirin has other positive benefits in addition to alleviating the pain of arthritis. For example, it may be effective for reducing the risk of a second heart attack. It may also be quite effective in reducing the risk of stroke in those who have had symptoms or actual strokes.

Most people take aspirin orally, but it can also be administered rectally through a suppository. Unfortunately, aspirin has a very short half-life, which means it gets out of your system fairly fast and thus must be taken frequently (approximately every four hours); many people find this quite inconvenient. One problem with aspirin is that many senior citizens have arthritis in addition to other medical problems that may be aggravated by aspirin. Some illnesses aggravated by aspirin are kidney disease, peptic ulcer disease, and stomach irritation. Coated versions of aspirin have become very popular recently, and we usually recommend them to our patients.

Other medications in the salicylic acid class include Disalcid, Dolobid, Mono-Gesic, and Salflex.

Propionic Acids   Propionic acids describe the class that includes such common medications as Aleve or Orudis. While these can be obtained over the counter, higher doses of the medication require a prescription. Also in this class is Motrin (ibuprofen), a medication many doctors regard with favor. It is considered to be relatively safe, effective, and low in cost. It can cause gastrointestinal irritation but seems to do so less often than does aspirin.

This class of medication, particularly the ibuprofen medications, has a relatively short half-life and rarely accumulates in the body. However, it can irritate the stomach and kidneys and should be used with caution. If you take other types of blood-thinning medicine, avoid this class.

Other medications in this class include Anaprox/Anaprox DS, Ansaid, Daypro, EC-Naprosyn, Naprosyn, Naprosyn suspension, and Oruvail. One new medication in this class is Naprelan, which can have a quick-acting effect and a long, sustained effect. We have had very positive experiences with Naprelan in our patients suffering from moderate to significant osteoarthritic pain. We have also found that this medication works not only for osteoarthritis but also for rheumatoid arthritis and general pain control.

Oxicams   The medication Feldene falls into the oxicam class. With careful monitoring, we find many of our patients do well on this medication, particularly those who need to be on medications for the long term.

Naphthylalkanones   The medication Relafen falls under the naphthylalkanone class, and it comes in either 500 or 750 mg tablets. This medication is for both osteoarthritis and rheumatoid arthritis, but because it's slower to take effect it's not considered a primary medication for pain management. The medicine seems to work best for individuals who have only mild pain and do not tolerate over-the-counter medications.

Arylacetic Acids   In this class of medications are a number of very potent medications, for example, Cataflam and Toradol. Toradol is available orally as well as in the form of an intramuscular injection, and it is frequently the nonnarcotic drug of choice in the emergency room for patients complaining of pain. Other medications in this class include Clinoril, Indocin, Indocin SR, and Tolectin. We are very pleased with a newer medication in this class, Voltaren XR, a long-acting Voltaren medication. In 100 mg tablets, it can be taken once a day, and it is relatively effective for pain from osteoarthritis and rheumatoid arthritis.

This class of medications has side effects similar to those of other anti-inflammatory classes, specifically stomach and kidney irritation. However, if monitored carefully, this class of medication can be fairly effective for intermediate and long-term use.

Pyranocarboxylic Acids   Lodine is a medication in this class. It comes in 200, 300, 400, and 500 mg tablets or capsules, enabling physicians to regulate the dosage to fit each patient. In addition, a newer extended-release LodineXL medication can be taken as two tablets in the morning, and it is very effective for osteoarthritis and rheumatoid arthritis.

Medications in this class can have side effects similar to those for other anti-inflammatories, although clearly the ease of dosing the Lodine medication makes this a popular choice for patients who need chronic pain management.

Exciting new research seems to show that individuals who use anti-inflammatory medicines on a relatively frequent basis may be at a *lower* risk for developing Alzheimer's Disease than those who don't take these medicines. Alzheimer's is a type of degenerative illness of the brain that affects thinking, mood, and behavior. We don't know what causes this disease; however, we're sure that more studies will provide additional information.

While all anti-inflammatory drugs have similar side effects, other medicines can help patients tolerate the side effects. Medicines such as over-the-counter stomach acid blockers (Zantac, Pepcid, Tagamet), prescription strength acid blockers, and even medicines that coat the stomach to prevent erosion of the lining can all be tried to help you tolerate prescription therapy, which is almost certainly the treatment your doctor will try first.

Analgesic Medications

Analgesic medication is simply another name for pain medication. This category is most popularly represented by the over-the-counter medication called acetaminophen. Known mainly by the brand name Tylenol, acetaminophen doesn't belong to an anti-inflammatory class, because it doesn't reduce inflammation. It is a simple pain medication only, but it can be quite helpful alone or in combination with anti-inflammatories. This is very useful for patients with mild to moderate pain.

Acetaminophen does not have the negative gastrointestinal side effects often found with anti-inflammatory medications. In fact, side effects from taking acetaminophen are relatively rare. High doses, however, have been known to cause liver damage, and extremely high doses can be lethal.

Other medications, such as muscle relaxants and narcotics, are often combined with acetaminophen for additional pain relief. For example, Tylenol #3 is a combination of aceta-minophen and codeine. Patients may also take acetamino-phen and other drugs separately.

Narcotics

Narcotics belong to a class of medication that is used to actu-ally numb pain. It comes from the Greek work *narcose,* which means "to numb." Narcotics are also known as opioid anal-gesics. These are medicines that ultimately stem from deriva-tives of morphine, although morphine itself is rarely used to treat arthritis pain.

The use of narcotics is a controversial issue. Just recently, federally approved guidelines were developed regarding the use of narcotics for nonterminal chronic pain, which previ-ously was considered taboo. In the past, physicians could have been fined for treating patients with narcotic medications unless dealing with a terminal or very acute illness or for treat-ment subsequent to surgery. Several pain management studies have revealed that patients are often undertreated rather than overtreated when it comes to chronic nonterminal pain; physi-cians' fears that they may be perceived as writing too many narcotic prescriptions is probably a major factor.

We attempt to use narcotic medications judiciously in our practice. Narcotics can have significant negative side effects and can also lead to addiction. However, we believe that nar-cotic pain management is an important adjunct in treating not only patients with acute arthritis pain but also patients with chronic pain. It's true, some physicians have used these medications inappropriately, but we refuse to "throw the baby out with the bath water."

Common side effects of all narcotic analgesics include dizziness, fatigue, impaired concentration, blurred vision, and nausea. Another bothersome and common side effect is constipation.

Narcotic analgesics are often given in pill form, although more potent versions can be injected. Oral versions of some narcotic medications (certainly not an exhaustive list) include Tylenol #3 and #4 (the number denotes the content of codeine in the medication), Darvocet N-100, Morphine Sulfate, Percocet, Vicodin, Lortab, and Hydrocodone. Codeine can also be given without additional components and as a straight codeine tablet.

There is also a long-acting narcotic medication, methadone. We find that methadone has a very minimal risk to be habit forming or addicting, and it is often an ideal choice for patients who have long-term painful conditions.

A newer pain medication on the market is Ultram (tramadol hydrochlorothide). This medication seems to be effective in relieving pain. It is almost as effective as the traditional opioids and it does not carry their high risk of chemical dependency. Ultram is actually a very weak opioid analgesic, but it has other properties that appear to block pain messages. It seems to act via neurotransmitters (chemical substances that carry messages between nerve cells). In particular, this medication seems to have a positive impact on serotonin, which we know from migraine pain management plays a significant role in blocking migraine pain. It also increases the effectiveness of another chemical messenger, noradrenalin. By activating these two chemical messengers, Ultram seems to block pain message conduction in the nervous system, and therefore pain is less intense.

Another pain medication is Stadol nasal spray. We feel that this is less effective for the subacute and chronic treatment of pain and rarely use it with our arthritis patients. This medication can be helpful when pain flares up and short-term relief is needed.

The pain patch is another form of medication that can be effective. Duragesic patch is one noted pain patch that can give pain relief for up to seventy-two hours without changing medication. It provides relief through the slow absorption of narcotic medication. Be careful to remove the old patch prior to placing on a new patch, to avoid toxicity. There is a moderate risk for habituation (habit formation) or even addiction with this type of chemical.

The implanted morphine pump is another form of delivering a narcotic, and this seems to be a much safer way to provide long-term narcotics while at the same time limiting a patient's access to the narcotic medication. The pump is actually implanted under the skin and is usually filled with morphine, like a reservoir, once a month. The pump has a computerized mechanism that can be set to give morphine at a constant rate or at a constant rate with extra doses at specified intervals. The morphine pump is quite expensive and is not without some risk for habituation or permanent narcotic condition.

Muscle Relaxants

A spasm is an involuntary contraction of the muscle. If the spasm persists for long periods of time, waste products are built up and released, leading to increased irritation of the muscle and ultimately pain. When muscles contract around a joint that is already inflamed, the result is both joint and muscle pain combined. Many physicians use muscle relaxants for spine and joint pains, particularly to reduce the spasms around the joints. Muscle relaxants can also reduce stiffness and the increased muscle tone that accompanies chronic joint inflammation. They are considered to be relatively safe.

The exact mechanism of how muscle relaxants work is unknown. It is thought to relax the muscles, although whether it works on the muscle itself, on the spinal cord, or on the pathways from the spinal cord to the muscle is not determined.

Drowsiness is one of the common negative side effects of muscle relaxants. Most patients would prefer to be awake and alert rather than drowsy. Some physicians feel that muscle relaxants have their most potent effect by producing drowsiness and subsequent sleep. During sleep or sedation, muscle tone is decreased in general, which may put the joints under less tension, thereby reducing inflammation. (We discuss insomnia in Chapter 8, certainly a common problem for those who have chronic pain syndrome.)

An additional side effect of muscle relaxants is that they can be fairly toxic. High doses are particularly toxic to the liver. As a result, muscle relaxant medications need to be carefully monitored.

There are many muscle relaxants on the market, including Flexeril (cyclobenzaprine), which is possibly the most frequently prescribed. Other common choices include Soma (carisoprodol), Parafon Forte (chlorzoxazone), Norflex (fenedrin citrate), Skelaxin (metaxalone), Robaxin (methocarbamol), and one of the oldest muscle relaxants available, Valium (diazepam).

Sleep Medications

As previously mentioned, patients with chronic pain often have a great deal of difficulty getting to sleep as well as staying asleep. Recent studies by the Sleep Disorder Society have found that when patients enter a deep sleep, there is a healing of their muscle, ligament, and joint pains. Conversely, patients who don't sleep have more pain. If the deep stages of sleep cannot be entered due to chronic pain, a vicious cycle occurs: the pain keeps them awake at night, leading to decreased ability to heal the joints and muscles, which leads to more pain.

In the past, "sleeping pills" were limited to treating patients with acute sleep problems, particularly if they were associated with an acute medical illness. However, we are now finding that chronic sleep disturbances can be equally devastating to a patient's daytime alertness as well as to general mood and outlook, energy level, stamina, and the patient's own subjective rating of his or her pain.

There are many kind of sleep medications. One simple medication is over-the-counter Benadryl. But before you rush to the nearest pharmacy and purchase a sleep medication, be sure that you discuss this first with your doctor. If you are on other medications, their combination with the sleep medication could cause negative side effects. It's also true that long-term use of over-the-counter sleep medications can actually lead to a rebound insomnia—thus leading to exactly the opposite goal that you had in mind.

You may have heard or read about melatonin, a substance that is readily accessible at most pharmacies and health food stores. Melatonin is a hormone that some people use to induce sleep. In humans, it is naturally produced by the pineal gland and appears to be involved in modulating various body functions, including sexual drive and reproduction cycles. Abnormal release of melatonin by the pineal gland may actually play a role in disorders such as anorexia nervosa and depression.

Melatonin that you can buy in stores has been called a "natural sleep aid," and some of our patients have reported very positive effects. However, you should be aware that dosages vary from one name brand to another. For example, one pill from the XYZ company may be equal to two from the ABC company. Always check the bottle if you switch brands!

Some people have found that melatonin has the opposite effect on them: it keeps them awake and may actually cause insomnia. Despite these problems, melatonin is a relatively safe and effective medication, and we have no qualms with our patients using it on a trial basis, as long as they carefully chart the results so we can monitor positive or negative effects.

Other sleep-inducing medications are the traditional sedative or hypnotic medications, such as Restoril or Halcion, and these act as muscle relaxants as well as sleep medications. In our practice, we have had very positive results with Ambien (zolpidem tartrate). This is an oral sleep agent relatively new to the market. It is available in 5 and 10 mg doses and can often produce the positive benefit of sleep without the "hangover effect" that is seen in some of the other sleep medications. There have been rare reports of negative side effects with the medication, although we have not observed any in our fairly extensive use of the medication.

Antidepressants

Patients with chronic pain—whether from migraines, back pain, or arthritis pain—all suffer a classic pain process that involves three components: physical, chemical, and emotional.

Chronic pain can be likened to a dripping water faucet. For the first few hours or days, the leaky water faucet is annoying, but it's not painful or uncomfortable. Over a series of days to weeks, however, it becomes uncomfortable and then painful; over weeks and months, it becomes torture. The water drop in the dripping faucet does not change. What changes is our ability to tolerate this dripping or the sound that the water drop makes. In essence, our pain threshold continues to lower and lower until finally we pass pain and move on to suffering, which is pain plus an emotional component.

There have been many explanations for this lowering of the pain threshold, but most neurospecialists who deal with chronic pain feel that the neuropharmacology of the nervous system changes, that chemical transmitters are at play, and that the chemical messengers are being irritated and depleted by a constant stimulation. This ultimately leads to not only the pain but also to a hidden depression, where all the signs of depression may not be obvious.

Depression is a common, predictable consequence of many conditions. Severe pain alone can cause the depression and despair that one sees with a chronic illness. Other aspects of a chronically painful state include the inability to maintain a positive self-image and the inability to perform routine activities that bring pleasure and joy. Often, individuals with chronic pain from osteoarthritis or rheumatoid arthritis are socially isolated, and this isolation can lead to emotional distress. In addition, the difficulty with sleep that individuals often experience feeds the chronic pain cycle.

Physicians who are comfortable treating chronic conditions, particularly chronic painful conditions, usually know that the depression from the chronic pain syndrome can be worse than the syndrome itself. This problem definitely needs to be addressed by doctors, and a number of medications have proven effective. In the past, such depression was treated with tricyclic antidepressants, such as amitriptyline, imipramine, nortriptyline, and desipramine. These medications have negative side effects, including extreme lightheadedness, dry mouth, weight gain, blurred vision, and in men, difficulty with urination. Also, heart palpitations and heart rhythm disturbances can occur. Other more effective medications have been found.

Over the years, there has been an explosion in antidepressant therapy. Many of the newer antidepressants have been found to be safe and effective, including Prozac (fluoxetine), Wellbutrin (bupropion), Zoloft (sertraline), Serzone (nefazodone), and Paxil (paroxetine). They seem to act on the serotonin reuptake inhibitors, allowing more serotonin to be effective in the brain; this lets the chemical messengers of the brain tolerate the "dripping faucet" better, thereby changing the suffering back to simple pain.

When antidepressants are effective, they will frequently raise patients' energy levels, resulting in less fatigue, more stamina, more endurance, and an improved outlook. This allows patients to return to their social settings, thus easing the problem of social isolation.

An additional newer medicine called Effexor (venlafaxine hydrochloride) has been efficacious. Effexor seems to block not only the serotonin but also the norepinephrine reuptake inhibitor. The result is that more serotonin chemicals and norepinephrine are available in the central nervous system. Individuals with chronic pain are often noted to be somewhat inattentive and easily distracted, leading others to think that these individuals are confused or have a memory impairment when actually the pain is blocking their attention and their ability to concentrate. The norepinephrine can act as a stimulant, producing increased mood, motivation, and vigor, as well as improving attention.

We have had a great deal of experience using Effexor, which comes in various dosages and has had many applications. For instance, we have found this medication to be extremely helpful in the medication management of adults with attention disorders (see our book *Adult ADD—The Complete Handbook*). When it comes to managing depression combined with decreased mood, motivation, energy, and stamina, we have found this medication extremely effective.

Cortisone Injections

We cannot discuss arthritis medications without mentioning cortisone, a true anti-inflammatory that is steroid in nature. This medication can often alleviate inflammation immediately and produce dramatic reductions in pain levels. Unfortunately, cortisone must be used sparingly, because it has significant negative side effects, including a loss of mineralization in the bones as it leeches away calcium and other minerals from the hard surfaces. Cortisone can also lead to fluid retention. In addition, if patients have a tendency towards diabetes mellitus (elevated blood sugar), cortisone injections can make this worse.

We use cortisone injections, locally as well as in the deep joints, and we have had some very good results. Nevertheless, this medicine should be used sparingly and with caution, and it cannot be used on a sustained basis. Prolonged usage could lead to kidney and liver damage or gastrointestinal distress. Patients on cortisone therapy, either by injection or in tablet form, must be watched very carefully. At the earliest sign of any negative side effects, cortisone should be tapered.

Combination Therapies

Physicians often use a combination of medications, such as a narcotic plus an anti-inflammatory, a muscle relaxant plus an anti-inflammatory, or an antidepressant plus a narcotic medicine. For example, if an individual is having difficulty with sleep and is experiencing a great deal of spasm because of joint pain and inflammation, then a physician may choose to use a sleep medication at night, an anti-inflammatory medication once or twice a day, and a muscle relaxant as needed for spasm.

Frequently, patients need "copharmacy" to treat various aspects of their pain. Despite the wonders of modern pharmaceuticals, one pill does not fit all. And trial and error with multiple medication is often necessary. We recommend to our patients that only one medication be changed at a time. While this might make good common sense, we are still surprised by how many patients we see who have been started on three (sometimes more!) medications at once—and then proceed to develop side effects. When we ask them if they can tell which medicine caused what side effect, not surprisingly they can't. We explain the pros and cons of copharmacy to all of our patients so they understand the possibility of a drug-drug interaction.

Weight Loss and Other Medications

We've talked about a variety of traditional medications used to treat inflammatory conditions and pain in this chapter. We also discuss several other medications in other chapters of this book. For example, many people with arthritis have problems with their weight; an estimated 70 percent of all people who have knee replacements are overweight people with osteoarthritis. Therefore, some people with arthritis could benefit from taking medications for weight loss, such as the new medicine Redux, which we discuss on page 111. In addition, we cover nontraditional medications, such as Pycnogenol and blue-green algae, in our chapter on nontraditional treatments in Chapter 5.

Of course, most people, including most of the patients in our practice, would prefer to live without medications. In the next chapter, we talk about many of the nonmedication and nontraditional therapeutic regimens available for the treatment of acute and chronic arthritis pain.

5

Alternative Therapy

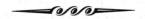

In earlier chapters, we've provided general information about arthritis as well as what to expect from a traditional physician visit and various medications that most traditional physicians use in treating arthritis pain. Now it's time to shift gears.

This chapter is for people who want to take an active role in initiating therapy for their arthritis pain. Particularly, it is for people interested in nontraditional treatments: healing touch therapy, relaxation therapies, biofeedback, diathermy (heat/cold therapy), acupuncture, and yoga. We will discuss homeopathy, tai chi, and electric stimulation therapy. In addition, we'll cover magnet therapy, which some experts consider a revolutionary approach to treating both acute and chronic pain as well as muscular complaints associated with arthritic conditions. We will also talk about natural therapies, in the form of herbs, natural ingredients, antioxidants, and nutritional supplements.

Therapeutic Massage

Therapeutic massage is often used to treat both chronic and acute arthritic pain and can be very effective in relieving muscle spasms. Massage increases the blood flow to the affected areas and also improves the removal of metabolic wastes through the lymphatic system. Sensory receptors in the skin and muscles are stimulated by massage to start healing areas that have felt "cut off" by chronic tension and pain patterns.

In addition, massage therapy often reduces or altogether eliminates the need for pain medication by stimulating the production of endorphins, the body's natural pain killers. Therapeutic massage prescribed by your physician can be very effective alone or in combination with other treatment plans.

There are many different types of massage. Neuromuscular massage is the type of massage therapy in which the muscles and the muscle coverings (the fascia) are released and relaxed through stretching and deeply stimulating the muscles. This is quite different from the relaxing Swedish massage that most people think of when they hear the word "massage." Swedish technique is a gentle form of massage that is done as much for relaxation as it is for muscle and joint pain relief. Both may have therapeutic benefits, but for arthritis pain relief, we prefer neuromuscular massage. There are numerous additional techniques of massage, and licensed massage therapists are always glad to review the various techniques with you.

Massage can hurt a little, however, and patients may feel some muscle soreness for a day or two after neuromuscular massage is performed. This soreness is the result of two processes: the accumulated wastes in the muscle tissue are now being manually released, and direct contact is made with the painful muscle spasm during treatment. This soreness is similar to what many people experience after strenuous exercise, and it will begin to diminish after the first few treatments.

After your massage session, drink as much water as you can stand. Water will help your body eliminate the released toxins. Also, apply an ice pack to the treated area for fifteen to twenty minutes frequently throughout the day—this will help reduce posttreatment soreness.

Craniosacral Therapy

Performed by holistic massage therapists, craniosacral therapy refers to a light touch and adjustment of the body from the base of the neck to the tailbone. The theory is that the flow of spinal fluid is altered, resulting in decreased pain in the spinal joints as well as diminished pain in the nerve roots along the spinal column.

Craniosacral therapy is not yet backed up by medical evidence, but some readers may find it a therapy worth investigating.

Hypnosis

Hypnosis is very different from the way it's depicted in the movies; your doctor will not use it to gain control of your mind for some nefarious purpose. Hypnosis is the voluntary achievement of a state of mind that can lead to pain reduction or even pain elimination. Hypnosis is difficult to initiate when a patient is suffering an acute attack of joint pain. However, patients can be trained to self-hypnotize and consequently modify their own behavior and appreciation of pain during these attacks. Most patients who have been trained in hypnotherapy can learn to stop short their joint pain when they feel an episode or attack coming on.

Hypnosis is also a form of focused attention. When it works, this therapy enables patients to shift the focus away from arthritic pain. People who are successful with hypnotherapy can actually learn how to alter the body temperature in their achy arms, legs, and joints, which in turn decreases pain. By changing the body temperature in the affected joints, they can "cool off" a hot or inflamed joint. They can also warm up a restricted, immobilized joint. In essence, they are using the body and the mind to perform a sort of heat and ice therapy—with no heat or ice.

Hypnosis takes time and practice to master. We encourage our patients to practice self-hypnosis in both the pain and pain-free state so that they will be able to use this therapy while they are in pain.

Breathing Techniques

You might assume that you already know how to breathe. But the truth is that proper breathing techniques are not as simple as you imagine, and when you are in pain, good breathing practices usually go out the window.

When you are hurting, it's natural to draw yourself in and not expand your lungs. This results in hyperventilating, which means you are not getting as much oxygen as you need in each individual breath. Another problem is that when you are in pain you often breathe much faster than normal. Breathing incorrectly can lead to poor oxygen circulation and can actually aggravate the pain attack. Good breathing techniques can reverse this pattern, but you need to learn them and practice them.

With focused concentration and attention to your breathing patterns, you can proceed to slow and deliberate breaths. Also, by attending to your breathing cycle, you can send the appropriate feedback information to the nervous system, so it will "reset" itself and relearn to breathe correctly. After a while, good breathing becomes unconscious and natural. A new bout of pain may cause you to lapse, in which case you'll need to practice your good breathing again until the problem abates.

Breathing and Pain

During an acute attack, chemical pain messengers are released in the brain. One of these messengers is adrenaline, which is the "fight or flight" chemical. When adrenaline is released, breathing usually becomes shallow and rapid. The diaphragm (the main breathing muscle) and accessory muscles become involved. These additional muscles are usually around the neck and shoulders, but they may also be in the chest wall and upper back.

If the joints are already inflamed, strenuously working additional muscles can lead to further aggravation of arthritis and more pain. Then, with greater pain, more adrenaline is released and the rapid, shallow breathing increases. We now have a pain cycle developing.

To correct and sometimes reverse this pathologic response, you need to concentrate on proper technique. Breathing deeply and correctly from the diaphragm enables you to avoid the use of accessory muscles, and it allows you to have a controlled respiratory pattern. Oxygen levels will be maintained, and lactic acid, waste products from rapid breathing, and accessory muscle use will be diminished.

Recently, we were called into the emergency room to examine a patient complaining of numbness in both arms. The ER staff thought that a stroke was a little unusual in a man forty three years of age, despite his risk factors of high blood pressure and two packs of cigarettes each day. After a careful history and physical exam and a review of the CAT scan of his brain, we asked the patient about stress in his life. He described a recent job loss and marital stress, and as he spoke, he was becoming more and more agitated. With this increased agitation, the arm numbness returned. His breathing rate increased, and he was hyperventilating.

The numbness in this man's arms was caused by his hyperventilation associated with stress—and with this rapid breathing rate, he was breathing out carbon dioxide and breathing in oxygen at a rate too high for his body to handle. We provided some breathing technique corrections and a referral to a psychologist especially skilled at teaching relaxation.

How to Breathe Correctly

Deep diaphragmatic breathing (deep breathing) exercises are best performed in a calm, quiet, and comfortable environment. Practice deep breathing techniques when the pain levels are at a minimum and not when you're in the midst of an acute arthritic attack. Breathe slowly and steadily, with a deep inhalation and a slow exhalation. While you are doing this, concentrate on feeling your abdominal muscles, to promote deep diaphragm breathing.

Often, deep breathing techniques are reinforced with biofeedback, temperature measurement, and muscle skin sensitivity readings to allow patients some objective verification of their improvement. Simply timing respirations per minute is a way to monitor breathing patterns. It is most important to find the right cadence and rhythm for you, as everyone's breathing patterns are slightly different.

Good breathing can be useful on a daily basis, at frequent intervals throughout the day. We encourage our patients to set aside a few minutes two or three times a day to practice deep diaphragmatic breathing. This is also a good way to take a break from life's hectic daily activities.

Progressive Relaxation

Progressive relaxation is a simple technique, and it's easy even for a novice. An extension of deep breathing, it actually involves all the muscles. The idea is that by contracting and relaxing individual muscles in a progressive fashion, from the head to the feet or the feet to the head, you can focus attention on particular areas and away from the sore and inflamed joints.

Here's how to perform progressive relaxation. Close your eyes and concentrate. Start with the toes, contracting individual toes and then relaxing them. Working your way up the body, concentrate on the feet, calves, thighs, and buttocks, then the trunk, hands, arms, and shoulders, and finally the neck and scalp. In each individual area, contract the muscles for ten to twenty seconds and then relax the area for thirty to sixty seconds.

Progressive relaxation isn't a quick fix for pain, but this technique can move the focus away from the chronic pain of the major and minor joints and on to the individual muscles that may be stiff or sore. Over time and with increased practice, this technique becomes simpler and simpler to perform, and it can actually lead to an overall body relaxation phase.

Guided Imagery

Another form of relaxation therapy is guided imagery. In guided imagery, the patient imagines a pleasant scene, such as floating on a cloud, drifting on the ocean, or relaxing in a calm, safe environment. This imagery triggers a positive feedback mechanism in the brain, allowing the release of certain chemical messengers. Those chemical messengers in turn cause the release of pain-blocking chemicals from the brain (endorphins and keflins), which provide pain relief.

One of our patients, Sandra, sought medical attention for her spinal arthritis pain, but she was particularly sensitive to traditional medications and constantly had gastrointestinal distress, to the point that she developed ulcer irritation. Sandra had been present at our public seminar on various techniques to treat acute and chronic pain, and she was intrigued by the prospect of treating her pain syndrome without pain pills.

Gardening was a passionate hobby for Sandra, although she had long since given this pastime up because of her stiff back, sore knees, painful ankles, and the arthritic changes in her hands and wrists. Yet she still enjoyed being in her garden, and we used this as the springboard for her guided imagery. We instructed Sandra to imagine dressing in her gardening clothes and getting out her gardening tools. We told her to imagine the smell of the garden and the feel of working through the dirt and planting fresh flowers. We then told Sandra to imagine her flowers blooming and to imagine the aroma the flowers would produce.

While this didn't work immediately, Sandra really enjoyed this exercise and was ultimately able to use it and expand on it as a form of relaxation and meditation. She would do her guided imagery for twenty to thirty minutes at a time, two and sometimes three times a day. Sandra reported a significant subjective improvement in her pain syndrome. Although her bone density studies and joint mobilization showed only minimal improvement, she reported that her suffering from the chronic pain was dramatically reduced.

Guided imagery, very much like hypnosis, requires practice. It's often best performed during a relatively pain-free interval, to allow the body to relax more fully and enable the mind to focus on the imagery technique.

Meditation

Like deep breathing, hypnosis, and guided imagery, meditation is a mental exercise that is quite helpful in altering the mind's ability to control the perception of pain. In addition, it is very helpful in redirecting the mind's focus away from the chronic pain state.

Meditation is done five to fifteen minutes per day, sometimes more frequently (if you are lucky enough to have more than fifteen minutes a day to spare). It allows the mind to relax, take a break, and actually focus on feeling better.

Meditation is effective not only in reducing the acute and chronic pain from arthritis conditions but also in reducing the general stress and anxiety that comes with a chronic pain state. By focusing your brain, you can slow your heart rate, alter your breathing pattern, and reduce the negative feedback to the brain. You can actually slow down your brain and produce more relaxing, soothing brain chemicals instead of stress chemicals. Your improvement in breathing allows increased oxygen and an increased energy flow.

There have been a number of research studies on the results of meditation. The recent success of Gregorian chant tapes indicates that you can come away from meditation encounters with improved energy levels, improved vigor, decreased fatigue, and improved feelings of self. Also, if you practice meditation on a regular basis, you may find that you sleep better and can cut back on unhealthy substances such as tobacco and alcohol. Most important, you're very likely to find a significant reduction in your arthritic pain.

Biofeedback

A relatively labor-intensive type of training program, biofeedback is often very helpful for individuals with moderate to severe arthritic complaints. The technique enables patients to learn how to lower their body temperature, pulse, and other body functions. Mastering this technique is quite demanding and requires a dedicated pattern of use. The patient usually interacts with a therapist and some form of equipment (such as a computer), which allows the patient to see objective results.

During biofeedback training, patients are instructed to think of various activities, settings, and conditions, both positive and negative. In this way, the patient is trained to use calming and soothing images and monitor how the heart, pulse, and breathing pattern slow down or to envision alarming, exciting images and observe how the heart rate, pulse, and breathing pattern speed up. Various auditory and visual signals—sound tones, the galvanic skin response measurement (measurement of skin electrical conductivity) displayed as a simple graph on a computer, and heart rate monitors—can guide patients' responses as they develop their abilities.

The goal for a person with acute and chronic pain is to achieve and maintain a slow, controlled respiratory pattern. Success at reaching such a pattern offers many benefits: improved oxygenation, improved circulation, and decreased stress chemicals released from the brain. Biofeedback allows a person to develop mental control over what previously were presumed to be involuntary processes in the body. We have all heard stories of meditation specialists who can slow their heart rate and breathing pattern to almost nonappreciable levels. While this is extreme, it does demonstrate how the mind can control the body.

We have recently received additional specialty training in a new form of biofeedback called EEG biofeedback. In this special kind of biofeedback, the patient is hooked up to an electroencephalogram (EEG), which is a brain wave monitor. Neurologists have known for some time that different brain wave patterns are associated with various mood states; brain wave patterns are noted to shift significantly throughout the waking and sleep cycle. In EEG biofeedback, patients are trained to address and control their brain wave activity. By obtaining a deeper, more harmonious rhythm to the brain wave patterns, they can reach a certain level of calm and a high level of pain control.

This type of training takes dedication and effort, but a cooperative patient can master it without too much difficulty. Once the patient learns key images or phrases to enter the synchronized EEG pattern, further EEG attachment to the device is not even needed. Our patients are very excited about our plans to institute EEG biofeedback. This technique is another method that empowers patients to become active participants in their health care and in their complete pain control.

Magnetic Therapy

Cleopatra wore magnetic bracelets, anklets, or amulets thousands of years ago to help with the healing process; she is only one of many who have believed in the power of magnetic therapy. Today, some people are convinced that magnets make them feel significantly better.

Magnetic therapy uses the concept of biologically effective magnets, not the simple north-south direction of magnetic polarity. According to this theory, negative polarity predominates and improves long-term healing.

Although we may not realize it, most of us have had a positive magnetic experience in our lives. For example, many of us have felt calm, refreshed, and restored when sitting by a quiet stream or brook, without the hustle and bustle of our daily schedules. One theory is that increased positive/negative ions surrounding these bubbling brooks or flowing streams in some way affect our energy fields, providing positive energy and restoring our sense of wellness. Similarly, when we sit in an oxygen-enriched environment, such as a forest, we seem to feel refreshed. One theory is that with the increased oxygen content, along with positive magnetic ions, we have a greater supply of oxygen-enriched energy coursing through our body, allowing us to have a higher level of wellness.

A Johns Hopkins treatment pain center study compared magnetic therapy for chronic pain to placebo therapy (there is no real benefit to a placebo except sometimes in the person's mind). While some individuals in placebo therapy improved minimally, people using the magnetic therapy showed a dramatic improvement. In addition, there were no side effects from magnetic therapy, thus making it an apparently reasonable choice for individuals who have tried and rejected traditional therapy.

Of course, not all types of magnets are free of side effects. For example, there is controversial evidence of negative effects stemming from high pulsating magnetic pollution and high-power transmission lines. These negative effects supposedly cause problems such as memory loss, headaches, changes in heart rhythm, and altered blood chemistry.

Those who have used applied magnetic therapy, in an appropriate fashion, have made some interesting and dramatic claims. Some orthopedic surgeons use magnetic technology in combination with traditional surgical intervention, obtaining nonunion bone fracture healing rates of greater than 80 percent—a very significant finding.

We don't think there is a single traditional physician who doubts the efficacy of magnetic science in regard to magnetic resonance imaging (MRI) scanners; physicians rely on these very powerful imaging studies on a daily basis (see Chapter 3 for more on MRI). Nevertheless, when the topic comes up of adjusting the magnet polarity of our bodies for healing purposes, skepticism abounds.

Many anecdotal stories, particularly from magnetic therapy companies, describe athletes who have increased their exercise endurance and weight lifting or weight training ability through the use of magnets. Other stories involve individuals who have tried and failed all traditional and many nontraditional therapies, who were then "cured" by magnets. While we are traditional physicians and understand that anecdotal stories do not equal scientific research, certainly we cannot deny the claim that many people improve dramatically with the assistance of magnetic therapy.

One version of magnetic therapy is to alternate the pressure points of the body using magnets. In this way, we are perhaps dealing with magnetic acupuncture or acupressure instead of the traditional manual or needle forms. A number of human and veterinarian trials show that this procedure actually provides relief for musculoskeletal as well as joint pain.

Articles in clinical orthopedic journals describe patients with failed prior lumbar fusions and chronic pain. A number of these individuals in the magnet use study had increased fusion benefits and reduced pain, with further studies suggested.

Some treatment studies have described using electric stimulation for facial pain. Patients treated with both magnetic therapy and electric stimulation therapy improved dramatically compared to those treated with only medications.

Magnets have been studied for their effect on neck and shoulder stiffness, low back pain, muscle pain, joint pain, and arthritic conditions. Individual effects have varied, but based on the location applied, the length of time that the magnets were used, and the patient's positive attitude, effective ratings for reduction in pain in either the neck, shoulders, back, or lower extremities ranged from 56 percent to 98 percent improvement in the subjective rating of the patient's pain. The magnetic mattress was reported to be particularly effective, and again no negative side effects were found.

Types of Magnets

Magnets come in all strengths and are marketed by many different companies. We have had success with Nikken magnetic pads. These pads come as small pads, for localized joints such as the wrists, or larger strips, to be placed on the low back.

Magnetic balls can be used for hand therapy, very much like traditional hand therapy for joint pain. However, with the healing power of magnets, people seem to find that their joints have increased flexibility and strength. In addition, pain relief appears to last for longer periods, even after brief sessions of therapy.

One double blind study tested the efficacy of magnetic belts, using many subjects suffering from low back pain. (In a double blind study, the subjects, and usually the doctors as well, are not told which treatment they are receiving; this is done to avoid any bias.) The patients who had no magnets, weak magnets, or placebos showed minimal improvement. The patients who received a high-field magnet belt reported marked improvement in their low back pain.

One of our favorite forms of magnet is a relatively low-cost item (as far as health care expenses go; about $65), called Mag Steps. These come as a large, oversized pair of shoe inserts that need to be trimmed to your foot's natural dimension, with a flat, smooth surface on one side and a bumpy surface on the other. Individual preferences will determine whether to wear these inserts with the bumps up or bumps down; there is no right or wrong way to wear them. They seem to improve stability, gait, and balance and also improve energy and stamina when worn for long periods. Some patients claim that Mag Steps have reduced their leg cramps, muscle spasms, and weakness.

Other magnet products include the magnetic bed pad (about $450) and a handheld magnetic massager. Rubbing the massager over the joints and muscles seems to increase circulation, reduce inflammation, and, most important, reduce pain.

We have discussed magnetic therapy with our traditional physician colleagues, who once described this as charlatan therapy. But the proof lies in patient satisfaction and patient improvement. We feel that we are treating a person with an illness rather than an illness in a person, and because this is one more type of therapy that enlists patients' full cooperation, making them a partner in their health care, its value is clear.

We've often found an added benefit of magnetic therapy. If patients are willing to go through the routine and trouble of applying magnets, they usually also take the time to attend to their body and to be aware of their joints. They also are more likely to take the time to focus on their problem and on a treatment or intervention.

Cryotherapy

Another therapy that has gained many patient advocates is cryotherapy. This is a very high-tech sounding word, but it simply involves the application of cold to painful areas. When you apply an ice pack, you're using cryotherapy. Our patients often ask us when to use heat and when to use ice. The answer is that it depends on the injury, complaints, and the time at which these injuries or complaints occur. The use of cold or heat must be tailored to each individual situation.

Applying cryotherapy for acute conditions with intense inflammation is very effective. The coldness closes blood vessels and leads to a reduction in the chemical products (cytokines) that start the whole inflammatory process. Penetrating cold ultimately reduces swelling. As swelling is reduced, muscle spasm is also reduced. Another advantage of using cryotherapy is that the cold can act as a deep stimulation, which ultimately blocks the pathways of the small pain fibers. This theory was originated by Melzak and Wall and was one of the initial cornerstone theories in pain management.

In addition to applying ice packs to the painful joint, you can perform ice massage, which involves gently moving the ice over your skin. There is also a technique called "spray and stretch," in which ethylchloride spray (a cooling/freezing surface anesthetic) is used on the muscles, and when the muscles are numb, the muscles, ligaments, and tendons are stretched. As the muscles warm up, the cool, numb sensation usually gives rise to a burning, warm sensation of the muscle and joint. This can be repeated periodically to increase mobilization and increase the range of motion of the inflamed joints.

Cryotherapy must be used in moderation; it is dangerous to leave ice on inflamed areas for more than twenty minutes. Making that mistake results in a reactive and negative secondary process: the blood vessels involuntarily open and the ice could cause blood vessel damage. If you perform cryotherapy on a regular basis, apply the ice pack for twenty minutes, then take it off for an hour and repeat this process to the affected joint.

Heat Therapy

The application of heat is a treatment for multiple processes, including joint pain and arthritis pain. There is an enormous market for heating rubs and heating creams, and nearly every day you can see a TV commercial espousing the virtues of deep heat and heating therapy (and a cream) to reduce pain.

The concept behind heat therapy is that heat opens the blood vessels, causing metabolic irritants to be carried away. Heat also nourishes the inflamed areas with nutrients. Ultimately, this leads to tissue healing. Heat also tends to increase the elasticity and flexibility of inflamed joints, tendons, and ligaments.

Moist heat—applied through special heating pads, hot showers, and whirlpool baths—tends to be more effective than the dry heat obtained from a standard heating pad. Often, the moist heat application is performed for twenty to forty minutes.

In general, heat therapy is a relatively safe, effective, and inexpensive treatment for the pain and stiffness of arthritis. We feel that heat therapy works better for chronic pain than for acute pain. In fact, if an injury is very acute, heat may actually make the situation worse.

Paraffin Therapy

While paraffin therapy, or hot wax therapy, is most effective for the fingers, it can also provide improvement for the wrists and elbows. This therapy involves placing the affected joint into the paraffin wax and letting the wax warm and soothe the muscles, ligaments, and tendons deeply. This process promotes increased vascular supply and increases the flow of nutrients into the inflamed joints.

Hot wax therapy should be used with caution, however, and under appropriate supervision, to avoid thermal burns or other complications that could aggravate inflammation.

Acupuncture

Considered for many years to be a nontraditional therapy, acupuncture has clearly come into its own. Most physicians appreciate the potential value of acupuncture as a safe, non-toxic, and relatively noninvasive way to manage pain. Prior to the advent of anesthesia, surgeons used acupuncture to block the pain of surgery.

Acupuncture, an ancient Eastern treatment, appears to work by releasing the body's own pain messengers. These chemical messengers (endorphins and encephalins) are our personal opiatelike substances. The same type of chemical messenger is released in the bodies of marathon runners, blocking the effects of their brutal running pace and allowing them to experience "runner's high."

Researchers don't know the actual neurophysiologic mechanism of pain relief, but they do know that the positive effects of acupuncture are blocked by the painkiller medications. This blockage indicates that the insertion of needles into various body energy pathways truly releases our brain's endorphins. A number of excellent books on acupuncture, as well as guides to the body's meridians for energy forces, are available.

We feel that acupuncture is very effective in providing pain relief, particularly for the major and minor joints of the extremities. Also, acupuncture can be very helpful for improving the body's gastrointestinal symptoms, as it seems to improve the contracting of the bowel and small intestine. There is also a reduction in nausea and stomach cramping. This is important, because patients with significant arthritis pain are often relatively sedentary, and constipation is a common complaint.

Yoga

Yoga is one of those unique activities that can have a very positive impact with minimal risk of any harmful problems. When yoga is performed in a relaxed, calm, and quiet setting, the patient can attain a state very similar to meditation. This allows the mind to focus away from the arthritis complaints and joint pain and on to other avenues.

There are multiple variations of yoga—certainly too many techniques and positions to mention or outline here. Briefly, the fundamental concept in yoga activities is stretching and flexibility, which allows the body to strengthen the major muscles, the supporting muscles, and the joints—the structural framework of the body.

By doing these stretching activities, the joints are able to bring in nutrients and extrude waste products from the joint space. This, in essence, lubricates joints and allows them to function in a more appropriate and pain-free fashion. Doing yoga on a regular basis can lead to increased range of motion, flexibility, reduced pain, and improvement in one's breathing pattern.

We caution our patients, particularly when they are starting a new yoga exercise regimen: not everyone has the full flexibility and range of motion that they would like or that they imagine they have, thus it's easy to overdo it. Obviously, very few of us are able to cross our legs behind our heads as a first step. Yoga, like any other form of exercise, takes time and patience to master. The benefits that one can obtain from this type of therapy, though, certainly make it worthwhile.

Homeopathy

Homeopathy is a discipline that was originally founded by German physician Samuel Christian Frederick Hahnemann in the late eighteenth century. The premise of homeopathy is that if a large amount of a medicine or substance produces a symptom or a negative/pathologic process in the human body, then small doses of this very same substance might actually cure the symptoms. For example, the drug belladonna is poisonous in certain quantities, but in minute doses, it can help with problems such as migraine headaches. We explain the role of belladonna in migraine management in an earlier book, *Migraine—What Works!* (Prima Publishing, 1996).

Modern science does not fully understand how homeopathy works. But we don't fully understand how aspirin works, either. The theory is that minute doses trigger the brain to "reset" itself, allowing the body's immune system to fight off the effects of the chemical, medicine, or substance causing the negative process in the body.

We point out to our patients who are interested in homeopathy that every chemical can have a different reaction in each individual patient and that patients respond in their own unique fashion. Therefore, it is important for patients to practice a trial-and-error approach under the guidance of an expert, just as they would with traditional medicines.

Space does not allow for a complete catalog of all of the homeopathic medications used or of the many natural herbs used to treat arthritis pain. However, we will mention that in minute amounts, chemicals such as arsenic, bryonia, and pulsatilla and herbs such as feverfew, nexpharmaca, geisemium, and senquinaria can be useful in treating arthritis.

Tai Chi

This ancient form of the martial arts came into prominence in the eighteenth century, when it was introduced in Beijing. Today, most people use tai chi more for its therapeutic value as an exercise rather than for its martial arts aspects.

The very nature of the patterned movements, performed in a slow and controlled fashion, improves circulation, increases range of motion, and loosens and limbers the joints. Tai chi also promotes mental relaxation and focused attention.

Many claims are made for tai chi. One is that it can retard and even cure some chronic conditions. While traditional medicine has no documented studies as to how (or if) this occurs, a number of anecdotal reports have attested to the benefits of tai chi. In our practice, we have found tai chi exceptionally effective for the management of chronic arthritis pain. It is also excellent for relaxation, anxiety reduction, and, more important, for gait and balance.

One of our patients, Bill, had a combination of spinal arthritis and Parkinson's disease, and he experienced severe difficulty standing and walking. This problem was attributed predominantly to his Parkinson's and was complicated by the fact that he had multiple levels of arthritis in the spine. Bill had tried numerous therapies, including exercise, strengthening, conditioning, water therapy, and gait and balance training. None of them seemed to provide any benefit, and he continued to weaken. Finally, almost as an aside, it was suggested that he seek tai chi training, since he was unable to do yoga or other forms of exercise.

At first, Bill had to do tai chi in a seated fashion. However, with diligence and practice, he improved a great deal. On a follow-up office visit, he astounded the entire staff by walking into the office without his cane. He was able to stand upright and demonstrated a marked improvement in his overall balance. There were psychological benefits to tai chi as well: Bill's mood, energy, and overall endurance and stamina had improved dramatically. This is a classic example of how self-directed therapy, requiring no special equipment, no special devices, and no additional expenses, can provide excellent therapeutic intervention.

Transcutaneous Electrical Nerve Stimulation (TENS) Therapy

The TENS unit is a small, battery-operated device that provides electric stimulation to the affected limbs and joints of arthritis pain sufferers. (Transcutaneous means "passing through the skin.") There are various ideas and rationales as to how the treatment works, some involving the release of endorphins, activating acupuncture meridian pathways, or overstimulation of nerve endings. Remember our earlier discussion on pain: basically, all pain messages must be relayed to the brain. If the stimulator produces an intense sensation of numbness and pressure, this numbness message may arrive at the brain first and effectively block the pain messages carried in on small fibers.

While TENS therapy may not be effective for acute exacerbations of joint pain, it has been proven to be a safe, relatively effective type of therapy for chronic painful conditions of the major joints. We have had patients with jaw joint arthritis and arthritis in the neck joints, hand, and finger joints who have used electric stimulation with excellent results.

If there is any electric rhythm disturbance in your body or if you have a cardiac pacemaker, then be sure to first discuss electric stimulation therapy with your physician. In addition, there has been some mixed literature on the use of electric stimulation on pregnant women; if you are pregnant or think you might be, ask your doctor if TENS therapy is appropriate. It comes as a battery pack, which looks very much like a pager with attached electrodes. These electrodes are attached to pads, which are applied to the muscles and joints that are inflamed. If you live in a hot climate or if you tend to sweat easily or have oily skin, then the pads may not stick well.

A new version of the electric stimulator is the Sol TENS, a handheld electric stimulator device. Our patients seem to like this device much more than the traditional TENS units. The Sol TENS has a probe that can pick up muscle and joint triggers and provide appropriate stimulation in a manual or timed fashion with a variety of intensities. This small device easily fits in a pocket or purse, and individuals feel comfortable using it rather than a medication, which may have side effects.

Although many of our physician colleagues were initially skeptical, they have seen that the electrical probe on the Sol TENS device does find the muscle trigger. After three or four stimulation episodes, the probe will no longer find these active hot spots—because they will be gone. Many patients have claimed significant relief from the use of this device, and their claims are backed up by findings of the Food and Drug

Administration that the TENS device works for myofascial and musculoskeletal pains. This is just one more example of new medical and biotechnology treatments that are becoming more user-friendly, effective, and appropriate for the injuries and illnesses they are meant to treat.

Mud Bath Healing

Mud or hot springs baths date back to the ancient Romans, who determined the siting of many of their cities based on the location of natural springs. Today, these hot baths are coming back into their own in the U.S. and elsewhere; Europeans, particularly Germans, value special baths in which peat bog or other substances help people with arthritis feel better.

While the actual explanation of why patients feel better after bathing or soaking in warm mud is uncertain, the practice is definitely booming. (A recent *Life* magazine story on integrative medicine depicts a mud-caked, Harvard-trained physician holding a peppermint sprig; this doctor is a strong proponent of mixing the two types of health care—traditional and holistic.) It appears that the heat of the mud, similar to the heat from soaking in a whirlpool, warms the muscles and ligaments surrounding the irritated joints. Various herbs are also used to increase circulation and provide relief.

Antioxidant Therapy

Oxidants are reactive oxygen species that are created by chemical processes. They may be harmful to body tissue and various cells. They seem to cause tissue damage and lead to degenerative changes. It has been postulated that by increasing antioxidants and consequently avoiding toxins, one can slow the aging process. More important for patients with arthritis pain, increasing antioxidants may slow down the inflammation and degeneration of damaged joints and cartilage.

A recent study in *Arthritis Rheumatology* (April 1996) reported that a high intake of antioxidant micronutrients, particularly vitamin C, reduced the risk of cartilage loss; it also reduced the risk of progression of illness in people with osteoarthritis. The report suggested that further studies be pursued to follow up this very important information.

Pycnogenol

Pycnogenol is one of the antioxidants that we have had a great deal of experience with, as discussed in our textbook, *Adult ADD—The Complete Handbook* (Prima Publishing, 1997). This is a trade name for a group of chemicals extracted from the bark of pine trees indigenous to the coast of southern France. Pycnogenol has been a folk remedy for hundreds of years and is a mixture of bioflavonoids. The beneficial effect seems to be the antioxidant properties of the bioflavonoids. This medicine has been touted by many who treat children and adults with ADD as a very powerful agent to help with concentration and attention. This natural remedy is also very helpful for individuals who have joint, muscle, and ligament pain. There are very limited negative side effects from Pycnogenol, and positive benefits have been cited in anecdotal stories.

Pycnogenol succeeds where some of the other antioxidants, vitamins, and minerals fail, and the reason for this has to do with our skin. The skin is the largest organ of the body, made of the epidermis (or outer layer) and the dermis (or inner layer). This inner layer is made up of elastic fibers—a comprehensive mesh network of elastic tissue. There is fatty and fibrous tissue beneath the dermis, a basic shock absorber that helps to protect our bodies. Collagen is one of the primary components of the dermis; it is a fibrous protein, made entirely of connective tissue, and it seems to thrive on vitamin C.

Pycnogenol enhances the positive healing effects of vitamin C and makes people feel better, often with much more energy and vitality.

Vitamin C

Vitamin C is a natural antioxidant, and it has proven very effective in the reduction of knee joint osteoarthritis. Dr. Cheraskin has published many books and feels that hyposcorbemia (the genetic inability to produce mineral forms of vitamin C) is the most devastating illness in the world. It leads to a breakdown of the immune system and connective tissue and leads to increased joint, muscle, and ligament pain.

Another proponent of vitamin C, Dr. Clemetson of Tulane University, reports that vitamin C is important to the treatment of all illnesses. Most of us remember learning in our high school history classes about sailors and travelers hundreds of years ago who suffered from scurvy before the advent of vitamin C pills. What we don't realize is that today we may be experiencing a low-grade form of inadequate amounts of vitamin C in our bodies.

If you don't have enough vitamin C, many problems may result. Joint and ligament problems can occur, and concentration is decreased (people low on vitamin C may be perceived as "scatterbrained"). A trial of vitamin C therapy is relatively simple, safe, and effective, and it won't lead to negative side effects as long as you have an adequately functioning kidney and liver system. We recommend vitamin C to all of our patients suffering from arthritic pain.

Vitamin E

Vitamin E has proven to be an effective antioxidant used by many traditional physicians, and it was recently touted as effective for reducing postexertional/postexercise myofascial pain. We prefer to use a dosage of 400–800 international units per day, which seems to be effective in muscle and joint pains as well as in reducing muscle cramps.

Keep in mind that vitamin E is one of the fat-soluble vitamins, and high doses can become toxic. Toxicity usually occurs in doses of over 2,000 international units per day taken for prolonged periods. We suggest that patients discuss vitamin E therapy with their physicians prior to initiating this type of regimen.

Folate

Folic acid is a vitamin found to play a role in neural defects in developing fetuses, particularly if the mother is folate-deficient. Moderate to higher doses of folate are considered protective. There is also some evidence that folate, with additional B vitamins (B_6, B_{12}), reduces certain levels of amino acids in the bloodstream that are correlated with heart disease. We recommend a one-a-day-type vitamin that includes folate, to avoid getting too much.

Vitamin B_6

We have had experience with the entire B catalog of vitamins. Vitamin B can be effective against attention disorder and migraine. Certainly a B vitamin combined with magnesium seems to be effective in many enzymatic processes throughout the body. We do urge caution, however, in using any of the B vitamins, because moderate to high dosages can lead to nerve irritation and nerve damage.

Beta Carotene

This antioxidant works in the conversion process to vitamin A and in general is considered safe and relatively risk-free. The theory is that this antioxidant works to protect cells from free radical damage; some people feel that beta carotene also prevents the onset of cancer. It can be effective in combination with other antioxidants in reducing chronic joint pain.

Minerals

There are many minerals that in very low to minimal amounts can be beneficial for your general health. Working closely with your body's natural healing sources, they have been touted to have positive benefits, including lowering cancer risk, increasing brain power, increasing athletic and general fitness performance, and protecting the skin.

Calcium and magnesium are two minerals that work in tandem and seem to be effective as protection against high blood pressure. We have also noted through our own research that magnesium seems to have a very powerful effect as a carrier for various vitamin B complexes. Calcium is recommended as a treatment or preventive mineral for osteoporosis, or bone loss (many patients with osteoarthritis also have osteoporosis). Calcium can be obtained in many forms; a simple check at the pharmacy or health food store will show you the various combinations available for both magnesium and calcium.

Chromium

Previously considered toxic, chromium was used primarily by automakers as the source for the shiny alloyed chrome. Automakers no longer use chromium, but today, nutritionists realize that chromium is a very potent ingredient for controlling hunger, increasing muscle tone, reducing body fat, and reducing heart disease and diabetes.

Chromium is widely available in tablets, capsules, liquid, and sublingual form. Many of our patients with arthritis have a condition of overweight syndrome or obesity (see Chapter 8), therefore this supplement may be very effective.

Coenzyme Q10

This vitamin-like substance was discovered in 1957. It was given this interesting name but actually could have been a vitamin. It appears that deficiencies of this chemical have been associated with various illnesses, including heart disease, hypertension, and joint degeneration. Co (Q substance 10) enzyme appears to stimulate and affect or modulate the immune system. Individuals claim that this chemical increases metabolism and therefore may be beneficial for weight loss, an effect similar to chromium.

Nutritional Substances

Under this category, we could include melatonin (see page 59). In addition, two chemicals—EPA (eicosapentaenoic acid) and DHA (docosahexaenoic acid)—are considered dietary fats. They are not "bad fats" and instead are very effective for improving cell membranes, increasing strength of nerves and muscles, reducing cholesterol, lowering blood pressure, and increasing circulation. These chemicals also have natural anti-inflammatory effects and are extremely effective in the use of arthritis. Some documented scientific research indicates cancer protection effects with these chemicals.

EPA and DHA are usually derived from the oil of cold-water fish as well as from a few plants. The plants that are particularly rich in these chemicals include evening primrose, borage, hemp, and black current. These chemicals are sold as liquids in oil-filled capsules, often combined with vitamin E. They come in many different strengths.

Acidophilus

Acidophilus is "good" bacteria often found in yogurt. The theory is that by maintaining sufficient numbers of healthful bacteria, particularly in the stomach and small intestines, other positive and protective substances can be absorbed better. Also, by maintaining a proper colony of your good bacteria, you effectively block out "bad" bacteria—dangerous species such as salmonella and staphylococcus.

Microalgae

These products are not isolated chemical compounds like vitamins but are rather concentrates. People take these because of their safety as well as their rich mixture of trace minerals, nutrients, vitamins, and antioxidants. The more significant forms, such as spirillum, chlorella, and blue-green algae, may contain additional nutrients that further enhance health. Recent literature has proven that phytonutrients (nutrients obtained through chemical and sunlight processes) may be cancer preventing and may have a positive impact on the immune system; broccoli and some Greek foods are rich in phytonutrients. In addition, they protect individuals from degeneration progression, particularly of the joints and ligaments, which is very helpful for arthritis sufferers.

One of our patients swears by blue-green algae. After taking blue-green algae, she was able to reduce her intake of prescription medications and later to avoid prescription medicines entirely. Indeed, this woman is a "modern miracle," according to her friends, family, and others in the medical community. Previously, she could not walk up or down stairs. Now she has boundless energy. Since no additional therapeutic intervention has helped with her chronic illness other than the blue-green algae, we must assume that this is the underlying factor in her improvement. While this is an anecdotal story, certainly further investigation should be pursued.

One school of thought regarding the benefits from blue-green algae and other phytonutrients is that vitamin B_{12} and other nutrients available from the algae may not be bio-available from another source; our bodies may require a nontraditional replacement, and the blue-green algae may play this role. Scientists know that in multiple sclerosis, a demyelinating disease (the nerve sheaths unravel), the B vitamins, magnesium, trace minerals, and essential fatty acids are all extremely important. Now, we may have another clue into chronic illness to demonstrate the need for phytonutrients that we can't obtain through traditional ingredients, natural food substances, or vitamin supplements.

It should be noted that blue-green algae, like any other ingredient that is ingested, may cause negative side effects; there have been reports of diarrhea and even liver slowing.

Caution is recommended in the use of natural, nonregulated, and noncontrolled substances.

Conclusion

In this chapter, we have looked at a wide variety of natural and nontraditional cures. If used in moderation and with the right attitude, the right physician, and support guidance, these remedies can be extremely effective in allowing you to find a treatment that works for you.

We encourage our patients to try various treatment regimens. This chapter is by no means a comprehensive guide to each and every one of the nontraditional therapies available. We have discussed just some of the approaches that we have taken with our patients to obtain the maximum benefit in therapeutic pain relief and to control and alleviate our patients' pain and suffering with their chronic arthritis condition.

6

Glucosamine Sulfate and Chondroitin Sulfate: The Whole Story

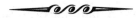

You have learned the basics of arthritis in previous chapters, and we have also discussed how successful treatment of arthritis can vary from individual to individual; Chapter 4 covered traditional drug therapy, and Chapter 5 covered alternative therapies. This chapter discusses glucosamine sulfate and chondroitin sulfate, regarded as a "miracle cure" in the book *The Arthritis Cure* by Jason Theodosakis, M.D. The purpose of this chapter is to outline the pros and cons of this combination therapy. We start by discussing exactly what these two chemical substances are and explaining the theory behind how and why they may be helpful. We also look at research findings, pro and con, on these substances.

The Normal Desire for Instant Pain Relief

Although we are traditional physicians, we are also acutely aware of human nature, being human and humane ourselves.

We know that when people hurt from the pain of a chronic illness, they will do virtually anything to feel better. We routinely ask our patients, as well as our professional colleagues, to keep an open mind when it comes to medications, substances, or any nontraditional therapy, because anything that might help a patient should at least be considered. Glucosamine sulfate and chondroitin sulfate are the latest drugs to give hope to patients seeking relief from arthritis.

Glucosamine Sulfate—What Is It?

Glucosamine sulfate is a naturally occurring substance found in large concentrations in animal joints. It appears to help increase cartilage components. It apparently achieves this increase by assisting the chondrocytes—the cartilage-making machinery of the joints that helps in the repair processes. Actually, glucosamine may help repair the breakdown processes in the cartilage of the joints. Joint cartilage breakdown can occur for a number of reasons, ranging from decay or deterioration from aging, to degenerative changes because of trauma.

As people develop arthritis due to wear-and-tear on the joints, they appear to have less glucosamine in their systems. In addition, the glucosamine that they do have seems to work less aggressively in repairing cartilage. The end result is that not only is the cartilage damaged, but the cartilage that remains seems worn out and is less effective as a shock absorber.

How *The Arthritis Cure* Doctor Sees It

In an analogy in *The Arthritis Cure,* Dr. Theodosakis compares the cartilage in a joint to a dense mesh of interwoven ropes. He says that this meshwork holds and attracts water, thereby allowing the cartilage to be spongy and fluid-rich and enabling it to act as a healthy shock absorber. The three things required in a healthy system include: (1) water, (2) a chemical substance called proteoglycans, which attracts the water and holds it in place, and (3) collagen, which holds the proteoglycans in place.

The theory is that the glucosamine seems to work by serving as a building block of the proteoglycans (the water holder). The more glucosamine there is, the more proteoglycans there are. And the more proteoglycans there are, the more fluid that can be held inside the cartilage tissue. In addition, some research shows that the more glucosamine there is, the more proteoglycans will be made by the chondrocytes.

In theory, therefore, the glucosamine not only helps build the machine, but also allows the machine to function more efficiently.

And What About Chondroitin Sulfate?

Chondroitin sulfate is the second substance recommended in *The Arthritis Cure* as the nutrient supplement therapy for arthritis symptom relief. Chondroitin is considered the counterpart to glucosamine.

Chondroitin sulfate is one of the many chemicals known as glycosaminoglycans or mucopolysaccarides. You may have heard of other glycosaminoglycans, which include shark cartilage, sea cucumber, and green-lipped mussel. All of these in various forms have been credited as effective for arthritis pain relief.

Returning to the earlier analogy of the meshwork, the system includes water, the proteoglycans that form the netting to catch the water, and chondroitin sulfate. The theory is that by acting as a long chain of repeating sugars, the chondroitin will actually "catch the water."

When we discuss the merits of glucosamine and chondroitin sulfate with our patients, we use the analogy of an upside-down umbrella. The glucosamine is the umbrella handle as well as the metal stays that spring out from it. The chondroitin sulfate, on the other hand, is the webbing that attaches to the metal stays, allowing an upside-down umbrella to truly catch and retain water. By attracting extra-cellular fluid, not only does the chondroitin sulfate theoretically maintain the high fluid content of the cartilage, but it also brings in additional nutrients and chemical substances that can nourish the cartilage.

Proper use of the joint causes compression and relaxation of the cartilage. The cartilage acts like a sponge, squeezing out waste products and bringing in nutrients. But to enable the extracellular fluid to nourish the cartilage and maintain its health, it's necessary to first catch it and transport it into the cartilage.

Pros: The Case for Glucosamine Sulfate/ Chondroitin Sulfate Treatment

Some scientific studies have outlined significant merits and benefits of the combination therapy. Other articles have outlined benefits from an individual therapy approach using only one medication or substance.

Looking at Supporting Studies

One of the more recent studies, by Müeller-Faßbender et al., revealed that after only two weeks there was significant pain reduction for patients in the group using glucosamine sulfate *and* for patients in the group using Ibuprofen, with the Ibuprofen group leading the way. By four weeks, there was a break-even point—both groups were about the same in efficacy. By eight weeks, the individuals using glucosamine sulfate passed the Ibuprofen group, reporting improved function and a decreased subjective rating of pain.

In another study, by Soldani and Romagnoli, the authors discussed the clinical value of glycosaminoglycans as well as the underlying physiologic function of these chemical substances. There was some positive benefit to glycosaminoglycans noted.

V. R. Pipitone's study suggested that chondroitin sulfate seemed to provide a protective benefit for cartilage in weight-bearing joints, such as the knees.

The literature supporting chondroitin sulfate and glucosamine sulfate dates back many years, including a number of articles from the 1970s and 1980s. There are also studies reviewing the use of oral glucosamine sulfate in treating osteoarthritis, and clinical investigations on the management of arthritis using glucosamine sulfate. A multicenter study and open investigation in Portugal in 1982 revealed benefits using oral glucosamine sulfate. There is also a reference to glucosamine sulfate and chondroitin sulfate in the book *Arthritis*, by Michael T. Murray, N.D. In this book, the author refers to many studies in the mid-1970s outlining the benefits of glucosamine sulfate.

Also notable is the clinical experience in Europe. Although the majority of studies cited in *The Arthritis Cure* are based on research from Asia, South Africa, and Europe, with only a handful of studies listed from the United States, these two supplements have mostly been used in Europe.

Not Many Side Effects

While there have been literally tens of thousands of individuals who have tried a glucosamine sulfate/chondroitin sulfate regimen, few significant side effects have been noted for this combination therapy.

It Works for Lassie

Some people think that the combination works well in animals. In the United States, this regimen has been used frequently in veterinary medicine. There has been a great deal of satisfaction among pet owners whose veterinarians prescribed a glucosamine sulfate/chondroitin sulfate regimen for pets suffering from joint pain.

Other Pluses

A recent article, "Put Out the Fire" by Jack Challam in *Natural Health,* cites numerous physicians arguing in favor of glucosamine sulfate as well as other traditional and natural cures. These supporters contend that the regimen has minimal risk for negative side effects. The true believers of this combination regimen also insist that not only will this medication reduce pain and joint swelling, but it will also attack the underlying inflammatory process and indeed effect a "cartilage cure."

We conclude our outline of "pros" with one that Dr. Theodosakis states: "the proof is in the lack of pain." His book cites numerous accounts of individuals who improved significantly, many quite dramatically. The examples and anecdotes described are truly amazing and would have to be considered nothing less than miraculous.

Cons: The Case Against Glucosamine Sulfate/Chondroitin Sulfate Treatment

As physicians, it is our sworn duty and responsibility to follow the first rule of medicine: Do no harm. Consequently, it is important for us to scrutinize any information about any medication before recommending it to our patients, families, or friends. Before rushing to proclaim glucosamine/chondroitin therapy as the cure, we think it's important to look carefully at the primary studies and determine their true merits.

Our Perception of One Study Differs

One of the studies cited in *The Arthritis Cure* was done in Milan, Italy, where researchers looked at eighty patients, all with severe arthritis. The patients were given glucosamine sulfate or a placebo (essentially a sugar pill).

After critically reviewing the results of the study, we were intrigued to learn that Dr. Theodosakis's conclusions varied drastically from ours. We realized that although 73 percent of the glucosamine group experienced a reduction in symptoms, compared with 41 percent in the placebo group, this high percentage really didn't mean much: 73 percent translates out to only 28 patients, and the 41 percent of the placebo group referred to 16 patients. So, essentially, 28 patients improved with the combination therapy, and 16 improved with the sugar pill. We are not impressed.

Also, the time for improvement in the glucosamine group was twenty days, compared with thirty-six days for those who received the placebo. In other words, the people who had the sugar pill did about as well as the people who took the glucosamine.

We asked ourselves: Why did sixteen out of forty patients improve after being given a sugar pill? What caused this improvement in nearly half the people in the study who were given a placebo? We contend that until this question can be answered, the therapeutic benefit of glucosamine as compared with a placebo does not constitute a glucosamine/chondroitin cure.

Also, if the patients really did have severe arthritis prior to treatment, how could they improve in thirty-six days to such a significant pain reduction? And with a sugar pill? We wonder what was going on here. Certainly, there must be some form of intervention that could play a role to alleviate this "severe arthritis" in individuals receiving a placebo.

A number of psychological studies have clearly demonstrated the powerful effect of placebo, particularly with the added factors of increased physician attention, greater clinical support, probable follow-up visits, and the patients' attention to their clinical symptoms over the course of the study. All these factors play a role in the patients' subjective complaints, particularly their subjective ratings of improvement of pain. The point is, were these psychological factors also playing a role in the individuals on the glucosamine?

Another study cited in *The Arthritis Cure* involved thirty-four patients, divided into two groups. This study seemed to rely on subjective rating, so it is difficult to assess individual objective improvement.

Dr. John A. Mills, associate professor of medicine at Harvard and a rheumatologist at Massachusetts General Hospital, has concluded that glucosamine sulfate and chondroitin sulfate are "probably harmless." He said in the "Harvard Letter" (August 1996), "You are better off seeing your doctor who can prescribe appropriate treatment such as anti-inflammatory or other anti-arthritic medicine." It is not uncommon for traditional medical specialists to espouse this viewpoint.

Possible Side Effects

Although we haven't seen serious side effects ourselves, some researchers are concerned about the possible side effects. Some scientific study reviews of these substances have pointed suspicious fingers toward the conclusion that these chemicals may lead to water retention. As a result, they may promote the production of proteins in the extracellular substance, which could lead to certain types of chemical breakdown enzymes in the extracellular substance of the joint. In turn, this problem could also cause irritation or degeneration of the joint. There is not yet enough scientific research in this vein, however, to know if we should really worry.

Do the Medications Actually Make It Through?

One of the strongest concerns about glucosamine sulfate/ chondroitin sulfate is the claim that they "get to the root of the problem," particularly with regard to inflamed cartilage and joints, and the allegation that they actually repair the joints. Traditional healthcare and nutrition specialists have pointed out that it is uncertain whether any of the glucosamine and chondroitin that you swallow is ever actually absorbed into the bloodstream. And even if it is absorbed, we don't know how much of it makes the trip all the way into the joint capsules and the extracellular matrix.

Some specialists have estimated that glucosamine sulfate administered by mouth can be absorbed up to 98 percent intact. But the estimates for chondroitin sulfate absorption are far lower, ranging from 0 to 8 percent, at most. Certainly, this is not a staggering amount, particularly when it comes to therapeutic benefit.

To compare glucosamine sulfate to chondroitin sulfate, we use the analogy of refined oil versus crude oil. There is certainly value in crude oil (chondroitin sulfate), but refined oil (glucosamine sulfate) can be used for many more purposes and is clearly much more effective and simpler to work with.

The Opinion of the Arthritis Foundation

Because of the popularity of the "cure" described in Dr. Theodosakis's book, the Arthritis Foundation has received plenty of calls, questions, and requests. So far it has taken a wait-and-see stance, but it is *not* recommending that patients with arthritis throw away their medications and take only glucosamine sulfate and chondroitin sulfate.

Physicians too look to the Arthritis Foundation for answers. When asked why it has not told the world about this "wondrous cure," the Arthritis Foundation's response is that neither it nor anyone else sees this combination treatment as a cure.

The Arthritis Foundation has announced that it is absolutely unable to recommend the use of glucosamine sulfate or chondroitin sulfate as a cure for arthritis. It classifies these chemical substances as "probably not harmful, but not considered scientifically acceptable as a treatment cure." Dr. Doyt Conn, senior vice president of the Arthritis Foundation, has stated that although there appear to be no significant negative side effects for this supplement regimen, scientific evidence has not supported it as a treatment to be recommended by the Arthritis Foundation.

If You Want to Try the Therapy, How Do You Start?

Assuming you have read other information on glucosamine/chondroitin therapy and understand the pros and cons discussed in this chapter—and your physician is unaware of any significant negative side effects—how do you start, and where do you get these substances?

The nutrient supplements come in an over-the-counter form, most often found at health food stores and nutrition supplement and natural therapy centers. It's also likely that these supplements will eventually become available in supermarkets and other outlets.

How Much Do You Take?

The dosage that has been most studied is glucosamine sulfate 500 mg (usually as capsules) three times a day. This can be taken with or without food; but if there is any nausea, stomach upset, or gastrointestinal distress, taking it with food should help alleviate that.

The chondroitin sulfate comes in 400 mg capsules; it too is often taken three times a day for a total of 1,200 mg per day. These dosage regimens are usually applied to individuals weighing 200 pounds or less. If a patient's body weight is more than 200 pounds, the dosage is increased slightly.

Looking at the Cost Factor

The cost for glucosamine and chondroitin varies moderately, depending on the brand of products you choose. On average, a forty-five- to sixty-day supply for glucosamine sulfate is approximately $50. A thirty-day supply of chondroitin sulfate is approximately $57. This amounts to approximately $450 to $500 per year for the glucosamine and $675 for the chondroitin sulfate.

This may not be a lot of money to some people, and yet to others it's a significant expense. Certainly, if cost is an issue, it's one mark for the negative side, especially if this expenditure removes healthcare dollars for more traditional—and possibly more effective—arthritis therapy.

Our Survey of Local Knowledge

We did our own survey of what area providers of glucosamine sulfate and chondroitin sulfate knew—if anything—about these substances. We called local pharmacies and food stores as well as natural therapy centers. At many of the national chain supermarkets, the pharmacist and staff in the health food section knew nothing about glucosamine or chondroitin sulfate capsules, including if they were available through the store or even if they were in stock. One national pharmacy gave us the cost but had no idea what dosage that cost referred to or how to use the medication.

Where to Go If You Try the Combination Therapy and It Doesn't Work

Let's say you try the glucosamine/chondroitin therapy. You follow the dosage carefully and you never forget a pill. You wait to get better and you truly believe that you will. But nothing happens. Do you lose hope?

Of course not. The therapy cannot work for every person. If you try it and it doesn't work, consider one of the many other traditional and alternative therapies described throughout this book. Consult your physician about any new ideas and discuss what you've learned in this book. Keep in mind that what works for your father or your cousin Susie may not work for you. So you move on and try something else.

What's the Bottom Line?

As with many healthcare issues, the glucosamine/chondroitin controversy is not black-and-white. There is a vast gray area of benefits, risk factors, and known versus unknown information. As we said in the beginning of this chapter, the American public has a thirst for treatment for chronic arthritis pain. The quick fix—the instant cure—is rarely readily available.

What we tell our patients is that sometimes it's a good idea to consider an alternative intervention. If you are interested in being an active participant in your healthcare, it is certainly reasonable to try the glucosamine/chondroitin regimen for a sixty-day period.

We have more than forty patients in our practice who have tried this regimen. Unfortunately, we cannot claim the success rates that Dr. Theodosakis does, although we do have a handful of patients who have reported improvement with the therapy.

We also have many patients who elected to discontinue use of this medication, although they seemed somewhat satisfied in that they tried it and understood what it was supposed to do. We have had very minimal complaints of side effects, with the most common being some stomach upset and some fluid retention.

We do not take the negative stance that the Arthritis Foundation takes, as we do feel that this combination therapy is a reasonable, relatively safe, and oftentimes effective therapy, at least in some of the literature. We point out to our patients that we truly do not know how aspirin works, yet we know that it is effective in heart attack prevention, stroke prevention, and anti-inflammatory therapy. Likewise, we feel certain that in the very near future we will have more scientifically controlled studies regarding the glucosamine/chondroitin regimen. We are also hoping for studies on additional combinations, such as anti-inflammatories combined with these natural nutrients and supplements.

Recall the concept of the combination lock theory that we discussed in the Preface. For our patients who have tried and been unsuccessful with this regimen, or who have not gained the relief that they expected, we point out that there are many types of therapies for arthritis pain relief.

Just as there are many types of arthritis, it would be unlikely and irrational to assume that there would be one cure-all. We have discussed more than twenty alternative therapies as well as many traditional ones; the following chapters discuss the importance of exercise and various healthful lifestyle changes. We feel that each individual, with his or her doctor, can find the right mix to open the combination lock of arthritis pain relief.

7

Physical Therapy

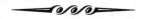

One of the most common traditional approaches to arthritis therapy is for physicians to prescribe physical therapy. A physical therapist (a person trained in anatomy and physiology) helps people with acute or chronic problems. In this chapter, we outline some of the various physical therapy techniques. We demystify physical therapy and what it entails, so you can understand what's being prescribed and the theoretical benefits.

The goal of all the therapies described in this chapter is to reduce inflammation, increase range of motion, and subsequently reduce pain. Some therapies cause a little bit of discomfort initially, because they break up muscle triggers (isolated areas of intense contraction of muscle fibers) as they increase the joint's range of motion. This discomfort is temporary and is usually worth it for the benefits you gain.

Ultrasound

Ultrasound therapy is generally performed by a physical therapist, physical therapy assistant, or therapy aide. This therapy directly reduces inflammation to the inflamed region by increasing heat and blood flow. Sound frequencies penetrate under the skin surface to achieve their mission; the closer to the inflamed joint the probe can get, the less sound frequency is required. Conversely, the more mass and muscle volume between the probe and the inflamed joint, the higher the sound frequency—the therapist has to "turn up the sound." After penetrating the skin, the sound waves act to warm the area, thereby increasing the circulation to that area of the body. Also, the sound waves act to directly "soothe" the inflamed muscles.

We've had very good results with this procedure, and it has helped our patients by reducing their pain and increasing their range of motion. However, it is a procedure that should be monitored carefully, to avoid muscle injury or burning.

Electrical Stimulation

Electrical stimulation is very helpful for alleviating pain associated with multiple joint and soft tissue injuries. This treatment increases circulation and the patient's range of motion by directly decreasing pain messages and inflammation. The stimulating probe sends out electric information, which sends pulses to nerve endings. This blocks the flow of pain messages to the nervous system, thereby producing analgesia. In addition, the electric probe can actually stimulate the release of endorphins (the brain's painkiller chemicals), and again pain is decreased.

Electrical stimulation is similar to TENS therapy (which we describe in Chapter 5), except it is performed using more potent (and expensive) equipment and under a therapist's supervision.

Another type of stimulation can lead to muscle reeducation. Electrical stimulation through electrodes placed on a muscle can actually strengthen the muscle, increase muscle tone, and allow the muscle to contract in a more appropriate fashion than previously. In this manner, the muscle is being reeducated. This technique is often used in combination with biofeedback, relaxation, or guided imagery. The goal is to improve muscle and joint function and ultimately alleviate pain.

Phonophoresis

Phonophoresis is a very simple and effective technique in which medications are applied to inflamed areas topically (applied to the surface of the skin). Then, an electric stimulating probe is used to drive the anti-inflammatory drugs and topical analgesics through the skin. The procedure is a direct application of pain-relieving and anti-inflammatory medication to the affected joints.

The probe can penetrate to a depth of five to six centimeters, which makes this treatment quite effective for inflamed joints and inflamed muscles. In addition, phonophoresis is useful for wound care, speeding blood flow and muscle healing following an injury or trauma.

Hot Packs

Contrary to popular belief, applying hot packs is more complicated than simply laying a heating pad on someone's inflamed joint (see also our discussion on heat therapy in Chapter 5). In a physical therapy setting, the procedure involves using a deep-heated pad with a special heat-absorbent substance in its center. This special heat-absorbent substance is warmed in a chemical unit called a hydrocollator, and caution must be taken to avoid muscle burns.

This technique is extremely effective in combination with other therapies, particularly those that increase blood flow and nutrients to the inflamed joints. Hot packs are applied for twenty to forty minutes, after which time the body's natural defense mechanisms kick in to try to block the positive effects of the heat. As a result, after that point, the benefit ends; continued application could make the problem worse.

Cryotherapy

Cryotherapy is the therapeutic application of ice, ice massage, or cold packs (see also our discussion on cryotherapy in Chapter 5). It can be extremely effective in reducing spasm occurrence, joint inflammation, and pain. Many people are confused by how ice should be used during the course of an injury. Our physical therapists believe that in most cases, ice should be applied to an acute inflammation and to acute injuries (or reinjuries) over the first forty-eight hours. We tell our patients to apply ice in the following way: on for twenty minutes and off for one hour, thereby allowing the blood circulation to work with maximum efficiency.

The ice closes down the small blood vessels, reducing blood flow and thereby reducing inflammation. However, if ice is left on for more than twenty minutes, the body's natural defense mechanisms will react, opening the blood vessels and actually causing a chemical freeze.

Myofascial Therapy

Myofascial therapy is the treatment of the muscle or, more correctly, of the muscle sheath that acts as its protective covering. In patients with arthritis, the muscles frequently become just as inflamed as the joints themselves. And once the muscle is inflamed, the cover or sheath becomes involved. This sheath has a very limited blood supply for nourishment. Therefore, it often stays inflamed due to lack of nutrients. The inflamed sheath will often restrict normal muscle function and range of motion (the muscle's protective mechanism to avoid even more irritation). Frequently, muscle triggers will develop, sending even more pain messages to an already inflamed and painful joint.

The trigger also prevents the full, natural range of motion and lengthening of the muscle. It weakens the muscle and leads to other muscles working to compensate, increasing the pressure on the already damaged and painful arthritic joint.

One of the more effective techniques performed in our clinic is called "spray and stretch," which we also describe in Chapter 5 (using ethylchloride). In this case, using a cryotherapy fluromethane spray, the muscle and joint are cooled and then stretched. Another useful technique is called trigger point massage: it starts with very light pressure using the fingertips, then slowly and steadily increases in pressure and tension, and ultimately allows the trigger to "release." When it does, the muscle can then stretch and function at its normal range of motion, with the muscle able to contract completely. This often completely alleviates the patient's painful muscle condition.

Traction

We sometimes recommend traction therapy for our patients suffering from arthritis of the cervical spine or neck. While it can be done at home, we often perform this therapy first in the office. In traction therapy, joints are actually, physically separated (slightly) to relieve the pressure on the joint; often this is done with spinal arthritis (as in neck or back traction). There are two types of traction therapy (plus variations): mechanical and manual.

In mechanical traction therapy, the physical therapist uses a mechanical traction device that can set the pressure and the speed of the pulling (or distraction) of the joints. Precise measurements are made of the amount of weight in pounds used to separate the joints. These settings can be reproduced from visit to visit to track patient progress. The traction pressure that is applied with a machine can either be constant (continuous) or it can be pulsing (intermittent); different patients respond to the different types. Time limits are set, to avoid any type of neck muscle injury. Often, after mechanical traction, patients experience complete relief of their neck pain as well as of their referred headache pain.

The second type of traction, manual traction, is limited by how long the specialist can actually separate the joint; also, there is no way to measure the pressure applied or to reproduce the session exactly at the next therapy visit. Nevertheless, we have observed manual traction combined with other therapies to be quite effective. It is a popular technique with chiropractic physicians, in combination with other joint adjustments.

Therapeutic Exercise

The underlying goal of any passive therapy program is to educate patients in the proper use of their joints and muscles and to allow patients to continue self-directed therapeutic intervention (passive therapy is therapy that is done *to* you or *on* you, as compared to active therapy, in which you do something, such as exercise). As we have explained elsewhere in this book, an overall healthful lifestyle and specifically a stretch program is key to your health. We've outlined for you in Chapter 9 very specific exercises to alleviate arthritis pain. Training is not easy, but you can learn through practice.

Therapeutic exercise under the guidance of a licensed physical therapist teaches you proper use of your joints. You'll also learn how to use resistance machines and how to perform toning, stretching, strengthening, and range-of-motion activities. In addition, the therapist will explain your individual weight limits, repetitions, frequency, and your time frame between exercise and circuit training (using various machines in a prearranged regimen, like at a health club). They'll use various machines and techniques to help you get a complete body workout in a safe, quiet, and controlled environment.

8

The Healthful Lifestyle

We have already discussed a variety of arthritis issues. It's also important to know that individuals with arthritis sometimes suffer from additional medical problems, all of which can lead to a downward spiral. One major problem is being overweight, and in this chapter we offer some recommendations to help with that problem. Also, you may be eating the wrong foods and/or you may be having trouble sleeping. We have advice for you that you can use right away. Remember: the downward spiral can be avoided!

If you suffer from severe knee joint pain, ankle pain, or hip pain (and sometimes from low back pain), you probably aren't eager to get out and exercise. As a consequence, your general metabolic rate slows down, your weight increases, your heart has to work harder, your lungs won't pump oxygen as efficiently, and your blood won't circulate as well. Your overall medical condition will start to deteriorate. In this chapter, we'll discuss the importance of exercise for everyone, particularly for the person suffering from arthritis pain. Keep in mind that most of the therapies we have outlined in this book are often best used when combined with exercise, proper body mechanics, general nutrition, and good lifestyle habits.

The Problem of Obesity

Obesity is a severe and at times devastating illness for many people in this country. If you weigh 20 percent more than your ideal body weight, you are considered "obese." If you weigh 100 pounds or more than your ideal body weight, then you are "morbidly obese."

Carrying around twenty or thirty extra pounds—or 100 extra pounds—places an extreme load on your body's musculoskeletal system and can result in damage to the muscles, ligaments, tendons, the soft tissues of the body, and, more significant for the person with arthritis, to the joints and joint capsules.

The popular TV health promotion and fitness guru, Richard Simmons, has a license plate that reads "YRUFAT" (why are you fat). Most patients suffering from arthritis know why they carry extra weight: it stems from the inability to exercise, and with this the pain and suffering continue.

Recent tests show that people who are overweight are at significantly higher risk for arthritis in the knees and are probably also at risk for arthritis in the hips and the hands. There is also a significant risk for additional serious medical problems, such as diabetes and coronary artery disease (narrowing of the arteries that flow directly through the heart muscle).

There is good news, though. Studies from the *American Journal of Clinical Nutrition* have demonstrated that weight loss can prevent the onset of symptomatic disease as well as alleviate symptoms you already have.

So if you are overweight and you have arthritis, what should you do? First, be aware that being overweight is a common problem for those suffering from arthritis pain. Then implement exercise and a healthful diet in your life—they are good ways to lose weight. Sometimes weight loss medications work well, too.

Fat-Busting Medications: Good and Bad

Over the past few years, there has been an explosion in weight loss medications. One popular and recent treatment involves the use of two prescribed medications (Fastin and Pondimin) in a nontraditional fashion; this is also called the "Phen-fen diet." This is *not* an approved weight loss regimen, and investigative reports have uncovered significant side effects.

One of the more dangerous side effects is the onset of what is called pulmonary hypertension, or increased artery pressure in the lungs, leading to backflow into the heart. This in turn leads to heart failure and critical complications. The problem can come without warning, and the condition must be monitored very carefully. Patients on these medications should be selected carefully by their doctors and should also be followed with blood pressure evaluations and laboratory testing.

Newer on the market is the medication Redux, which is the first medication formally approved by the Food and Drug Administration for weight loss. This medicine affects the serotonin chemical mechanism of the brain, leading to appetite and hunger suppression. It may also have positive effects on energy and mood and possibly on attention. Redux produces a slow and steady weight loss, which allows you time to learn correct nutritional habits. Redux costs about $2 per day for appropriate weight loss. We have had some very positive effects in our clinic with this weight loss medication.

You Are What You Eat

We've all heard of the chicken soup remedy as a cure for the common cold. Now scientific research is showing that

chicken soup and many other simple dietary staples are leading the way in improving arthritis pain. In one study, a Harvard teaching hospital created a "chicken soup" of collagen
and protein extracted from chicken breast bones combined in
a weak vinegar solution. They tested it on patients with
arthritis, and it made them feel better.

In another case, Dr. Norman Childers found that by elimi-
nating foods of the nightshade family (such as tomatoes,
potatoes, eggplant, peppers, and tobacco) from his own diet,
he alleviated his arthritis pain. His theory was that alkaloids
in these foods consumed in low doses over a long period of
time built up and led to additional inflammation and irritation
of the joints. He also felt that these agents would inhibit normal cartilage repair in damaged joints.

Michael T. Murray's book *Arthritis* has an extensive section on diet and supplements, including theory on how foods
can have both a positive and negative effect on an arthritis
sufferer's pain. In his book, Murray, a naturopathic doctor,
emphasizes the role of antioxidants and nutrients (which we
discuss in Chapter 5).

Do you remember when Mom told you to eat all your
broccoli and other green leafy vegetables? Guess what—she
was right again! It turns out that fresh fruits and vegetables
are high in antioxidants and in essential fatty acids, which is
the good stuff that your body needs to run all the chemical
processes that occur millions of times a day.

Mental Alertness and Your Diet

In Chapter 11, we discuss the relationship between chronic
pain and depression. But what about the relationship between diet and depression and being mentally sluggish?

A new branch of study, called nutritional neuroscience,
basically states: You are what you eat. This means you feel
good or bad based on what you eat, and you are either sharp
and alert or dull and sleepy based on what you consume.

A research study concluded that animals fed high concentrations of essential fatty acids were more energetic, learned faster, and exhibited less aggressive behavior than those not on the same enriched diet. In another case, a human study looked at mood and diet and found that individuals on an "American" diet (you know it: fast food, high in cholesterol, low in fruits and vegetables) were noted to be significantly more depressed and rated their energy level as much lower than those who ate a balanced diet.

Did you ever stop to wonder how Mom knew so much? Do you recall her telling you that fish is "brain food"? Well, it turns out that freshwater fish is extremely high in essential fatty acids (again, the good stuff that our bodies desperately need), so Mom was right once again. Eat your fish: think quicker, have more energy, improve your mood, and—oh yes, feel better with less joint pain!

We've compiled a handy chart, much like the one we use for our migraine headache sufferers. This chart lists foods to eat and foods to avoid. It is meant as a guideline only.

Vitamin D Levels

A number of recent articles have discussed dietary intake with regard to serum levels of vitamin D and how they relate to the progression of osteoarthritis. An article in *Annals of Internal Medicine* (September 1996) reveals that low serum levels of vitamin D and a low intake of vitamin D appear to be associated with an increased risk for osteoarthritis of the knee.

As nutritional general practitioners have known for some time, normal bone metabolism relies heavily on the presence of vitamin D, which is derived largely from your diet or from your skin's exposure to ultraviolet light.

Decreased systemic levels of vitamin D may have a negative effect on the body, resulting in such conditions as poor calcium metabolism, a breakdown of bone density and bone matrix, and decreased bone formation activity. Therefore,

Table 8.1 THE ARTHRITIS DIET

Food Group	Foods Okay to Eat	Foods to Limit
Beverages	decaffinated coffee and tea, alcohol (1 to 2 oz. per day), natural fruit juices, noncarbonated beverages, water	caffeinated drinks
Milk	soy milk, rice beverages	cow's milk, whole milk, buttermilk
Dairy products*	nondairy cheese, nondairy ice cream, yogurt, cottage cheese	all dairy products
Meat/meat substitutes	most cold-water fish (such as salmon, sturgeon, whitefish, bass, and perch)	liver, red meat, shellfish, herring, sardines, mackerel, anchovies
Bread/bread substitutes	whole grain cereals, homemade pasta (made with natural ingredients), bagels	brewer's yeast, homemade bread with yeast, chips, French fries, waffles, pancakes, cornbread
Fruits	one cup per day of: cherries, blueberries, grapes, dates, figs, apples, bananas, melons, or raisins	honey, sugar, jam or jelly
Vegetables**	No limit: cabbage, garlic, endive, lettuce, radishes, spinach, turnips, watercress	tomato, celery, chicory, cucumber, potato, peppers (except black pepper)
	In moderation: artichokes, asapargus, bean sprouts, beets, broccoli, brussels sprouts, carrots, cauliflower, eggplant, greens, mushrooms, okra, onions, rhubarb, sauerkraut, string beans, squash, zucchini	

Table 8.1 THE ARTHRITIS DIET *(continued)*

Food Group	Foods Okay to Eat	Foods to Limit
Miscellaneous	flaxseed oil, linoleic acid, chicken soup, nuts (flaxseed, canola, pumpkin seed, walnuts, sunflower seeds), soy	nuts (almonds, Brazil, cashews, macadamia, peanuts, coconut)

*Try complete dairy elimination from your diet. Chart your health, and introduce dairy products one at a time to monitor their effect on your health.

**Try juicing your vegetables.

low levels of vitamin D may lead to poor tissue healing, poor bone density, and even fractures. There are new medications that can help the body absorb and store vitamin D to avoid these problems. Fosamax, Calcimar, and Didronel are just a few of the many medications available. Patients on these medications should be selected carefully and should be followed with blood pressure evaluations as well as laboratory testing of bone density.

Complicating this equation is the fact that people who already suffer from arthritis may have more inflammation and also more erosion and degeneration of the bones and joints than if they already had "soft bones." Studies appear to support the finding that the arthritic condition along with a poor intake of vitamin D is a bad situation; in this case, vitamin D intake should be increased.

Vitamin C

Studies have shown that people with arthritis enjoy improvement by moderately increasing their vitamin C intake. (We discuss vitamin C therapy in Chapter 5.) Simple diet modifications may indeed be part of the puzzle in preventing arthritis progression in certain individuals.

Sleep Well, Be Well

Patients who suffer from severe arthritis pain often experience great difficulty falling asleep and maintaining a proper sleep cycle. We feel strongly that sleep is part of the healing process. Recent studies revealed that during deep stages of sleep, test subjects began to heal their muscles, tissue, and joints. Unfortunately, we have also documented through EEG sleep studies that people with chronic arthritic pain have a lot of trouble entering that deep, restorative sleep.

We have often heard, "If I could just get a good night's sleep, I know I would feel better." This is actually true, because a positive sleep cycle restores many physiologic functions of the body. In fact, that's why we have to sleep—because our bodies need it.

If you have insomnia or trouble staying asleep or waking up too early, your restorative process is often impaired. You feel listless, lethargic, and fatigued during the course of the day, which plays a negative role with your arthritis pain. Because you feel so tired, you have less energy to do activities and, therefore, you do less. You have slower metabolism, and you gain weight, feel more fatigued, and do even less. This is the beginning of the deconditioned and downhill cycle—a cycle that certainly needs to be interrupted.

The American Sleep Disorder Foundation has eloquently stated that some people may actually acquire a "sleep debt." People will go for days or even a few weeks of getting too little sleep, whether by half an hour or two to three hours. Ultimately, that sleep debt needs to be repaid. If it is not, then the individual starts to rapidly deteriorate with regard to mood, energy, and stamina, with increased pain, decreased alertness, and ultimately increased muscle discomfort. This lack of sleep has been found to play an important role in the disease called fibromyalgia, a muscle disorder.

Before you can correct this problem, you must identify the cause. Is it the pain alone that is keeping you up? Could it be chemicals or foods you ingested before going to bed? Or maybe it's lifestyle stress. Maybe your sleep environment is simply not hospitable to sleep.

It may sound strange, but one of the most notorious triggers for insomnia is sleep medication. While sleep medicines may work for a few days, most of them are meant to be used short term. Using sleep medications on a regular basis can lead to a "rebound phenomena," or a secondary insomnia, which is very difficult to treat.

Specialists who deal with sleep disorders often recommend a comprehensive sleep cycle evaluation to help determine the cause (or causes) of one's sleep deficit. This includes a careful history as well as a clinical assessment of a patient's sleep cycle in the sleep laboratory. Sometimes, if the sleep debt has not been repaid or has been repaid only partially, the sleep clock or day/night cycle is off by a few hours. This is an important concept to understand and is best discussed with a sleep specialist.

We provide some very simple and basic guidelines for patients suffering from sleep disturbance, including the following:

- Do not consume any caffeine or stimulant medication close to bedtime—say, within about two hours before you want to fall asleep. Some experts go further, recommending complete avoidance of caffeine at any time, as this can act as an irritant to the nervous system.

- Avoid alcoholic beverages prior to sleep time. While the idea of a nightcap or "just something to help me get to sleep" may be attractive, the alcohol irritates, inflames, and depresses the nervous system, leading ultimately to a rebound phenomena, which awakens your nervous system within a few hours.

- If you absolutely cannot sleep, then get out of bed. We recommend that our patients do something else rather than lie in bed agonizing over the fact that they cannot sleep. This simply leads to frustration and anxiety, which leads to an additional sleep dysfunction.

- Do not take little naps during the day. If you are not sleepy at nighttime because you have rested throughout the day, then you won't be able to fall asleep in an appropriate fashion. We do allow some of our older patients to take a thirty-minute to one-hour nap in the midafternoon, when cortisol levels are low (that is the adrenalin chemical in our body that keeps us awake, which seems to ebb at approximately three o'clock or four o'clock in the afternoon). By limiting a nap in this fashion, individuals do not destroy their routine sleep cycle.

- Do not go to bed angry, upset, or stressed. This sounds simple, but it still surprises us how many people describe tossing and turning through the night, agonizing over the day's business events, social events, and so on. By doing this, they clearly do not give their minds a chance to rest and are blocking their bodies' natural restorative processes. It is easy to say "get it off your mind before you go to bed," but it is certainly not always easy to do. Nevertheless, keeping this in mind should ultimately help with a positive sleep cycle.

Now that we have talked about things not to do before sleep, here are a few simple suggestions on how you *can* fall asleep:

- Work on and practice the positive relaxation techniques we have discussed earlier (see Chapter 5). They can be quite helpful for relaxation and can initiate drowsiness, restfulness, and ultimately sleep.

- Make sure your sleep environment is a positive and restful one for you, one where you can be comfortable. If possible, avoid loud noises, bright lights, and intermittent or periodic sounds. Some people find it helpful to turn on some sort of soothing sound, such as the crash of ocean waves, the noise of a tropical rain forest, and so on, to act as masking or "white noise."

- Discuss your problem with your physician or pharmacist and ask for suggestions and guidance. Medications you have been taking for a long time may be accumulating in your body, being poorly metabolized or simply building up, causing a problem with your sleep cycle. Be sure to communicate to your physician that you are having a sleep cycle problem. Without knowing about your problem, your doctor cannot make suggestions to improve your cycle.

• Feel free to discuss with your physician other sleep-inducing agents besides standard prescription pharmaceuticals. There are reports that some supplements, such as vitamin B3, calcium, and magnesium, as well as many herbs are helpful for sleep initiation. Valerian root and passionflower are two herbs with minimal negative side effects. In addition, melatonin is a natural aid for reducing pain and providing a positive sleep cycle (we discuss melatonin on page 59). Cautious use of this supplement may be very helpful in alleviating sleep distress.

Exercise Should Rule

We feel very strongly that exercise is not just useful for arthritis but is actually the fountain of youth—the magic cure for multiple medical processes.

In January 1995, we hosted a community-wide, free, day-long public seminar on exercise and aging at the Ritz-Carlton Hotel in Naples, Florida. We sponsored seventeen physicians, who all spoke about their specialties and how exercise ultimately could reduce negative processes from the natural aging condition.

Prior to the seminar, we had been touting exercise as a therapeutic benefit for strength, flexibility, endurance, stamina, pain reduction, and increased energy and vitality. Some traditional physicians were a little skeptical at our fervor. Yet when these doctors prepared for the conference (attended by over 1,000 community members), some were shocked to discover that the traditional research in their areas of special expertise had *all* shown that exercise was beneficial.

One experienced oncologist discovered that exercise reduced the risk for gastrointestinal cancer and breast cancer. A neurosurgical colleague found that exercise seemed to improve healing rates, reduce postoperative pain, and improve the patients' subjective rating of overall improvement following surgery.

Psychiatrists and psychologists at our seminar reported that exercise improved memory, attention, recall, naming, language, and judgment. Individuals who were challenged cognitively over a long period of time actually did better, were able to maintain their faculties, and had less confusion. People who were asked to use their minds continuously in a challenged fashion were less likely to develop dementia.

The cardiologist who spoke at the seminar was aware that exercise was helpful but was surprised to find out just how helpful it can be in preventing heart attacks, reducing blood pressure and cholesterol, and increasing energy and general fitness.

We felt the community was treated to a very thought-provoking and interesting seminar, but more important, we think that the physicians involved were forced to realize just how powerful exercise can be.

Our Patients Are Proof

Every day in our exercise and spine rehabilitation centers, we hear from patients whose doctors had told them it was "only arthritis" and they would have to live with it, and after following the exercise regimen we recommended, how much better they feel. These individuals previously could not dance, play golf or tennis, go for a long walk, or engage in social activities. After enrolling in a planned, patterned exercise program, their overall arthritic pain decreased, their general medical conditions improved, and they were back to enjoying a healthful lifestyle.

We often ask our patients to enroll in a formal strengthening, stretching, and flexibility program, under supervision. We've been backed up by an article in the *British Journal of Rheumatology*, in which a study revealed that people trained in an at-home exercise program, without formal exercise intervention, did not do as well and did not continue in the program for as long as those who did engage in a formal program.

Even after a directed program, some people are still unable to do aggressive activities. We often start these individuals in a chair exercise program. Marching in place while sitting in a chair can be simple, safe, and effective, and it can improve circulation and the regular breathing pattern. After a week or two, when this is no longer a challenge, we add weights—and we like to use the expression "Soup is good weight." Pick up a full soup can and do small bicep curls while you are marching in place in a seated position. This exercise is easy and can improve cardiovascular fitness.

When biceps curls combined with marching are no longer a challenge, we have our patients do arm lifts, lifting the soup cans from their side directly up to midshoulder height and then back down again. They can progress to overhead soup can lifts combined with marching in a chair. If they can tolerate this, then they usually can proceed to additional intervention, typically at a fitness club or a wellness center.

Water therapy is ideal for our patients with arthritic complaints. The water's buoyancy lifts them up, so there is no joint pressure, alleviating pains in the hip, low back, knee joints, and ankle joints. Walking in the water is very effective therapy; it is based on the principal of progressive resistance (used in Nautilus exercise programs): the faster one walks in the water, the more the water pushes back and the more progressive the resistance becomes. A twenty- to thirty-minute brisk water walking session in the shallow end of the pool, back and forth, can be an extremely challenging aerobic workout. Inexpensive devices such as water wings and arm attachments can also be used to do arm exercises in the shallow end of the pool, to increase upper body strength and coordination as well as to reduce joint pressure and pains.

Whatever Exercise You Choose—Do It!

The most important concept in exercise—more than where you do the exercise, who supervises you, or how much you do—is "Use it or lose it." If you don't do the activities, your muscles will shrink and bones and joints will become swollen and inflamed; certainly there will be no gain of flexibility, strength, stamina, or endurance.

On the plus side, the more you use your muscles, joints, ligaments, and limbs, the better you will be. Some physicians have argued in the past (incorrectly) that continued exercise would actually lead to deterioration of the knee joints, ankle joints, hips, and low back. An article in the *Journal of the American Geriatric Society* (January 1996) shows that musculoskeletal injuries rarely occurred during exercise, and indeed no major injuries were noted in the study. Moderate-intensity, stationary exercise cycle and strength training appeared not to exacerbate joint symptoms in older adults.

In addition, a study published in the *Arthritis and Rheumatology Journal* (January 1996) reveals that vigorous running activity did not increase musculoskeletal pain with age. Indeed, particularly in women, there was a reduction in pain. Also, vigorous physical activity was associated with low subjective ratings of pain compared to sedentary positions.

Exercise is once again proven to be an antidote for arthritic pain as well as for many other medical conditions. In the next chapter, we demonstrate some very simple and direct stretching exercises to allow you to get started on a home therapy program.

9

Stretch Your Health

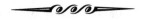

The exercises that follow can provide the means to safely increase muscular strength, endurance, range of motion, and flexibility of the lower and upper body. When performed regularly, these exercises will strengthen the soft tissues that stabilize and support the spine, pelvis, trunk, shoulder girdle, and lower extremities. In addition, exercises that will help strengthen the wrists, hands, and fingers have been included. By doing these exercises, you can reduce joint pressure, increase range of motion of inflamed joints, and alleviate arthritis pain and suffering.

Most of these exercises should be done with resistant bands in order to offer a progressive resistant exercise program. There are varying levels of resistance. Once you can complete 3 sets of 15 repetitions without pain or discomfort, you may consider increasing the resistance of the band.

The available resistance levels usually include medium, heavy, and extra heavy. Exercise bands are available through local pharmacies, or you may order a band by calling 1-800-844-7880.

Helpful Hints for Using a Resistance Band

- Inspect the band before each exercise session for any nicks, tears, or worn areas that may have occurred from use.
- Protect your band from tears or punctures by keeping it away from sharp objects. Remove rings before using and be cautious of long, sharp fingernails.
- Store your band in a dark area away from direct sunlight. Occasionally sprinkle the band with talcum powder.
- Use a bow or a knot to tie the band. Always make sure the knot is secure before you exercise.
- Untie and flatten the band before storing. The band can be easily untied.
- You may wish to wear protective clothing such as socks or pants to prevent the band from pulling at your leg hair.
- Do not stretch the band more than 10–15 feet. Over-stretching the band may result in serious injury.

The exercises outlined in this chapter may not be suitable for you. Use your own good judgement and consult a health care professional prior to engaging in the exercises outlined herein. The information is not intended as a substitute for individualized evaluation and medical advice. *Do not* do any exercises your doctor or therapist has told you to avoid.

─────── BEFORE YOU BEGIN ───────

Warm Up!

A good warm-up prior to exercising is essential to prepare the body for increased activity and to reduce the chance of injury.

An active warm-up increases the temperature of the tissue surrounding the joint and aids in improving muscle flexibility.

The warm-up should consist of maintaining a continuous activity such as walking, bicycling, or marching in place for 5–10 minutes, followed by gentle stretching exercises. In addition, stretch after each strength-training session to allow your muscles to adequately recover, which will help to prevent muscle and joint soreness.

Stretch Your Health Exercise Guidelines

- The exercises illustrated in this chapter should be practiced three times a week to achieve optimal strengthening of the desired muscle groups and to gain the maximum benefit in alleviating joint pain. Allow one day of rest between strength-training sessions.

- Body alignment is critical, especially with standing exercises. Stand with feet shoulder-width apart, contract the abdominals, square the shoulders, and relax the knees. Maintain a good posture throughout the exercise. Your eyes should remain open at all times to help maintain balance.

- When performing each exercise, work the muscles throughout the full range of motion. Do not lock the joints.

- *Do not hold your breath.* Breathing should be slow, rhythmical, and under control. Slowly exhale as you move into the first or most difficult phase of the stretch. Breathe slowly as you hold the stretch. Inhale as you return to the starting position.

- Stop exercising immediately if you get chest pain, shortness of breath, or become dizzy or sick to your stomach.

- Perform each exercise in a controlled and slow manner. Do not allow your limbs to bounce or jerk with movement. Control all movements throughout the complete range of motion. You should resist the band throughout each exercise.

- Gently move an inflamed joint (one that is hot, red, swollen, or painful) through its range of motion.
- *Do not* stretch past the point of discomfort. Stretch to the position where you feel a mild tension in the muscle, hold for 1–3 seconds, then relax. Stop the exercise before you reach the point of pain.
- Use a stable object such as a chair or countertop for balance when performing lower body exercises.
- Strengthen all the major muscle groups and perform an equal number of exercises (repetitions) on each side of the body. This will decrease your chance of developing muscular imbalances.
- Begin each exercise with 1 set of 10 repetitions.
- Add 5–10 repetitions as the exercise becomes easier.
- Exercises performed with improper technique and/or resistance will not facilitate strengthening of the desired muscle groups. Please refer to the illustrations frequently to ensure proper form.

To Reduce
Shoulder Arthritis and Bursitis

Shoulder Flexion

Position   Sit on the edge of a chair or stand on a firm surface with the band held at hip or waist height.

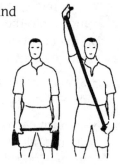

Movement   Raise and extend one arm toward the ceiling, keeping the elbow straight. Point thumb toward the ceiling. Hold for 1–3 seconds at the farthest point. Slowly return to starting position. Repeat on opposite side.

Position Stand on a flat surface with the band under right foot. Arm to side, hold the band with your right hand at hip level.

Movement Raise one arm toward the ceiling. Keep elbow straight and thumb toward the ceiling. Hold for 1–3 seconds. Slowly return to starting position. Repeat on opposite side.

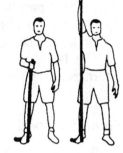

Position Stand on a flat surface with the band under both feet. Keep a slight bend in the knees and elbows. Arms to the side, hold the band at hip level.

Movement Raise arms toward the ceiling. Keep elbows straight and thumb toward the ceiling. Hold for 1–3 seconds. Slowly return to starting position.

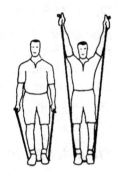

Shoulder Extension

Position Stand on a flat surface with the band held at waist height.

Movement Extend left arm back, past the hip. Keep left elbow straight. Hold the right arm at waist level. Hold for 1–3 seconds. Slowly return to starting position. Repeat on opposite side.

Position Secure the band to a stationary object at shoulder level. Stand facing the wall with both arms extended out at shoulder level, palms toward the floor. Grasp the band.

Movement   Lower arms to side, slightly past hips. Squeeze shoulder blades together. Keep elbows straight. Hold for 1–3 seconds. Slowly return to starting position.

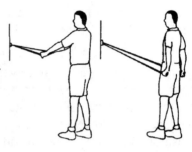

Shoulder Abduction

Position   Stand or sit on the edge of a chair. Hold the band at hip or waist level. Point thumb toward the ceiling.

Movement   Raise one arm away from the side of the body. Keep elbows straight. Hold for 1–3 seconds. Slowly return to starting position. Repeat on opposite side.

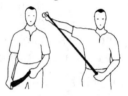

Shoulder Adduction

Position   Secure the band to a doorknob or stationary object. Stand with the right hip facing the secured band. Loop the band around your right arm.

Movement   With your right hand, pull the band across the front of the body. Keep elbow straight. Hold for 1–3 seconds. Slowly return to starting position. Repeat on opposite side.

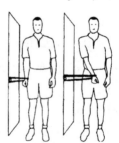

Shoulder Horizontal Abduction

Position   Secure the band to a doorknob or stationary object. Sit with side of body to door. Loop the band around the wrist of the arm farthest from the door.

Movement Using the arm farthest from the door, pull the band across chest and out to the side. Hold for 1–3 seconds. Slowly return to starting position. Repeat on opposite side.

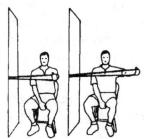

Position Secure the band to a wall hook or stationary object at slightly above shoulder level. Stand facing the wall with feet shoulder-width apart. Extend arms toward the wall, holding them at shoulder level. Palms face inward. Grasp the band.

Movement Pull arms back, maintaining elbows at shoulder level. Squeeze shoulder blades together. Hold for 1–3 seconds. Slowly return to starting position.

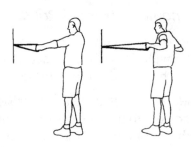

Shoulder Horizontal Adduction

Position Secure the band to a doorknob or stationary object. Sit with side of body to door. Grasp the band in the palm of the hand closest to the door. Palm faces away from door.

Movement Using the arm closest to the door, pull the band across the chest to the opposite shoulder. Hold for 1–3 seconds. Slowly return to starting position. Repeat on opposite side.

Position   Secure the band to wall hook or stationary object slightly above shoulder level. Stand with back to the wall and with feet shoulder-width apart. Extend your arms out to the side with elbows bent. Palms face inward.

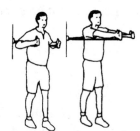

Movement   Pull the arms forward, extending elbows. Hold for 1–3 seconds. Slowly return to starting position.

Modification   This exercise may be performed using one arm at a time.

Shoulder External Rotation

Position   Secure the band to a doorknob or stationary object. Sit with side of body to door. Grasp the band in the palm of the hand farthest from the door. Palm faces door.

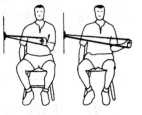

Movement   Pull the band across body and out to the side using the arm farthest from the door. Keep elbow bent and pressed to side of body. Hold for 1–3 seconds. Slowly return to starting position. Repeat on opposite side.

Shoulder Internal Rotation

Position   Secure the band to a doorknob or stationary object. Sit with side of body to door. Grasp band in the palm of the hand closest to the door. Palm faces away from door.

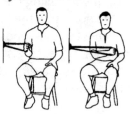

Movement   Pull the band across body to stomach, using the arm closest to door. Keep elbow bent and pressed to side of body. Hold for 1–3 seconds. Slowly return to starting position. Repeat on opposite side.

Shoulder Shrugs

Position   Stand on a flat surface with the band 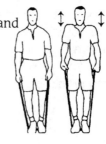 under both feet. Keep a slight bend in the knees and elbows. Arms to the side, hold the band at hip level.

Movement   Shrug shoulders, lifting toward the ceiling. Hold for 1–3 seconds. Slowly return to starting position.

Chest Exercise

Position   Sit or stand with feet shoulder-width apart. Loop the band around each palm. Hold arms in front of body with elbows slightly bent. Palms face the floor.

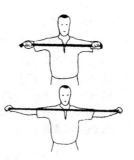

Movement   Pull the band outward, across the chest. Maintain a slight bend in the elbows. Hold for 1–3 seconds. Slowly return to starting position.

Seated Row

Position   Sit on a firm surface with your legs in front of you. Loop the band under the balls of both feet. Grasp each end of the band, keeping elbows straight. Palms face down. Maintain good posture by keeping your back straight and tightening the abdominal muscles. Keep a slight bend in the knees.

Movement   Leading with the elbows, pull both ends of the band toward the torso. Keep arms close to the sides of the body to squeeze the shoulder blades together. Hold for 1–3 seconds. Slowly return to starting position.

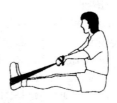

Caution   Proper body alignment is important with this exercise. Do Not lean forward when returning to the starting position. Contract the abdominals and keep the back straight. Maintain proper breathing technique.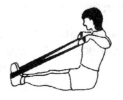

TO REDUCE HIP, THIGH
AND SACROILIAC PAIN

Hip Flexion

Position   Secure the band to a wall hook or stationary object (such as a table leg) at mid-calf level. Stand on a flat surface with your back to the wall. Loop the band around one foot. Hold leg in a 90-degree angle. Maintain a slight bend in the knee of the supporting leg.

Movement   Bring leg forward and up to hip level. Hold for 1–3 seconds. Slowly return to starting position. Repeat on opposite side.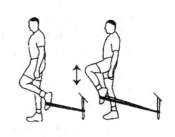

Position   Secure the band to a wall hook or stationary object at ankle level. Stand on a flat surface with your back to the wall. Loop the band around the ankle. Begin with legs together.

Movement   Extend leg forward, keeping knee straight. Maintain a slight bend in the knee of the stationary leg. Hold for 1–3 seconds. Slowly return to starting position. Repeat on opposite side.

Hip Extension

Position   Secure the band to a wall hook or a stationary object at ankle level. Stand on a flat surface facing the wall. Begin with legs together.

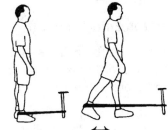

Movement   Extend leg back, maintaining a slight bend in the knee. *Do not* lean forward. Hold the stretch for 1–3 seconds. Slowly return to starting position. Repeat on opposite side.

Hip Abduction

Position   Secure the band to a wall hook or stationary object at ankle level. Stand with side of body to the secured band. Loop the band above the ankle on the leg farthest from the secured band. Begin with legs together.

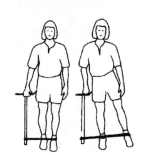

Movement   Slowly lift leg with the band out to the side, maintain a slight bend in the knees. Hold for 1–3 seconds. Slowly return to starting position. Repeat on opposite side.

Hip Adduction

Position   Secure the band to a wall hook or stationary object at ankle level. Stand with side of body to the secured band. Loop the band above the ankle on the leg closest to the secured band. Extend the leg with the band toward the secured object. Maintain a slight bend in the knee of the opposite leg.

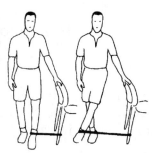

Movement   Slowly bring leg with the band across body in front of the stationary leg. Hold for 1–3 seconds. Slowly return to starting position. Repeat on opposite side.

Hip Internal Rotation

Position   Sit on a firm surface with the band around a chair or table leg. Loop the band around the ankle.

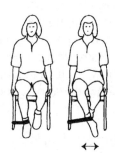

Movement   Keeping thigh flat on surface, lift foot with the band slightly and move lower leg toward the center of the body. Hold for 1–3 seconds. Slowly return to starting position. Repeat on opposite side.

Hip External Rotation

Position   Sit on a firm surface with the band around a chair or table leg. Loop the band around the ankle.

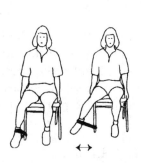

Movement   Keeping thigh flat on surface, lift foot with band slightly and move lower leg away from the center of the body. Hold for 1–3 seconds. Slowly return to starting position. Repeat on opposite side.

——————— To Reduce Knee Arthritis ———————

Knee Flexion

Position   Secure the band at ankle level to a stationary object. Sit on a firm surface, facing the secured band. Loop the band around ankle in a figure 8 pattern.

Movement   Bending from knee, pull leg with band back. Hold for 1–3 seconds. Slowly return to starting position. Repeat on opposite side.

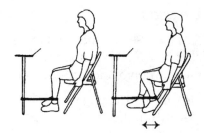

Knee Extension

Position   Secure the band at ankle level to a stationary object. Sit on a firm surface, with your back to the wall. Loop the band around ankle in a figure 8 pattern.

Movement   Extend leg with band, straightening the knee. Hold for 1–3 seconds. Slowly return to starting position. Repeat on opposite side.

─────── **TO REDUCE ANKLE ARTHRITIS** ───────

Inversion

Position   Secure the band to a stationary object. Sit on a firm surface with the band to your side. Loop the band around the mid-portion of foot.

Movement   Holding your heel on the floor, slowly move the forefoot with the band in toward the center of the body. Hold for 1–3 seconds. Slowly return to starting position. Repeat on opposite side.

Eversion

Position   Secure the band to a stationary object. Sit on a firm surface with the band to your side. Loop the band around the mid-portion of the farthest foot.

Movement   Holding your heel in place, slowly turn the foot with the band away from the center of the body. Hold for 1–3 seconds. Slowly return to starting position. Repeat on opposite side.

Plantar Flexion

Position   Sit on a firm surface with legs out in front of you. Loop the band under the balls of one or both feet, with toes pointed toward the ceiling. Grasp both ends of the band. Maintain good posture by keeping the back straight and tightening the abdominal muscles. You may lean against a wall for back support. Maintain a slight bend in the knees.

Movement   Point toes toward the floor. Hold for 1–3 seconds. Slowly return to starting position.

Doris Flexion

Position   Secure the band to a wall hook or stationary object at ankle level. Sit on a firm surface, such as the floor, with your leg(s) extended. Loop the band firmly around the fore-foot (just below the base of the toe joints) of one or both feet, toes pointing toward the ceiling.

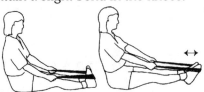

Movement   Pull foot towards shin. Hold for 1–3 seconds. Slowly return to starting position. Repeat on opposite side.

EXERCISES FOR
INFLAMED FINGER JOINTS

Hand, finger, wrist, and arm pain is often a result of chronic arthritis pain. If you have been diagnosed with this, or any other painful condition of the wrist, hand, or fingers, the following exercises will help strengthen the muscles of the hand and arm.

Start slowly so you won't cause additional pain and inflammation. Begin with the finger exercises. When you are capable of completing 2 sets of 15 repetitions without pain or discomfort, continue with the hand, wrist, forearm, and elbow exercises. These exercises are best accomplished using a small strip cut off the end of the band or a thick rubber band.

Finger Flexion

Position   Wrap the band around an individual finger or all the fingers. Hold the end of the band with the other hand.

Movement   Pull fingers in toward the palm. Hold 1–3 seconds. Slowly return to starting position. Repeat with other fingers on the opposite hand.

Finger Extension with Thumb Abduction

Position   Wrap the band around an individual finger and thumb or four fingers and thumb.

Movement   Slightly cup hand, and spread fingers and thumb apart. Hold for 1–3 seconds. Slowly return to starting position. Repeat with other fingers on the opposite hand.

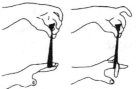

Finger Abduction

Position   Wrap the band around two adjacent fingers or all of the fingers.

Movement   Spread the fingers apart. Hold for 1–3 seconds. Slowly return to starting position. Repeat with opposite hand.

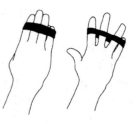

Thumb Extension

Position   Wrap the band around the fingers and thumb. Palm faces the ceiling.

Movement   Move the thumb outward from the hand. Hold for 1–3 seconds. Slowly return to the starting position. Repeat with the opposite thumb.

Thumb Opposition

Position   Wrap the band around the base of the thumb. Hold the ends of the band with the other hand.

Movement   Move thumb with the band up and over to touch the tip of the little finger. Hold 1–3 seconds. Slowly return to starting position. Repeat with the opposite thumb.

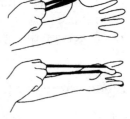

--- **TO REDUCE WRIST PAIN** ---

Wrist Flexion

Position   Sit with forearm on a table or chair arm, holding the right wrist slightly over the edge with the palm up. Hold

the other end of the band under the right foot or with the
opposite hand at knee level.

Movement   Raise your right hand
toward the ceiling, holding the
forearm on the table or chair
arm. Hold for 1–3 seconds. Slowly
return to starting position. Repeat
with the opposite hand.

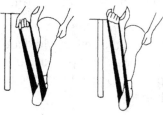

Wrist Extension

Position   Sit with forearm on a table or chair arm holding the
right wrist slightly over the edge with the palm down. Hold the
other end of the band under the right foot
or with the opposite hand at knee level.

Movement   Raise your right hand
toward the ceiling, holding the forearm
on the table or chair arm. Hold for 1–3
seconds. Slowly return to starting position. Repeat with the opposite hand.

Ulnar Deviation

Position   Sit with right forearm on a table
with the palm facing down on the table. Stabilize the band with the opposite hand.

Movement   Move your right hand out away
from the body. Hold for 1–3 seconds. Slowly
return hand to starting position. Repeat
with the opposite hand.

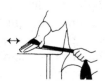

Radial Deviation

Position   Sit with right forearm on a table or chair arm, holding the wrist slightly over the edge, thumb pointing toward

the ceiling. Stabilize the other end of the band by tying it to the table leg or chair arm.

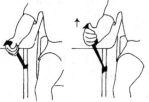

Movement   Raise your right hand toward the ceiling. Hold for 1–3 seconds. Slowly return to starting position. Repeat with the opposite hand.

To Reduce Elbow Arthritis

Elbow Flexion

Position   Sit in a chair without arms. Secure the band at knee level to the right chair leg. Loop the band around the right forearm in a figure 8 pattern. Palm faces the ceiling.

Movement   Pull your right forearm toward shoulder, bending at the elbow. Hold for 1–3 seconds. Slowly return to starting position. Repeat with the opposite arm.

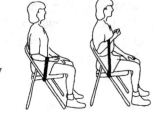

Elbow Extension

Position   Sit in a chair with right elbow bent. Secure the band around the right arm of the chair. Grasp the band with your right hand, palm facing down.

Movement   Straighten your right elbow. Hold for 1–3 seconds. Slowly return to starting position. Repeat with opposite arm.

Pronation

Position   Sit in a chair with your left forearm resting on left thigh. Loop the band around left hand, palm facing up. Stabilize the other end of the band under one foot.

Movement   Rotate your left palm down toward the floor, holding the forearm on the thigh. Hold for 1–3 seconds. Slowly return to starting position. Repeat on the opposite arm.

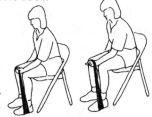

Supination

Position   Sit in a chair with your left forearm resting on left thigh. Loop the band around left hand, palm facing down. Stabilize other end of the band under left foot.

Movement   Rotate your left palm up toward the ceiling, holding the forearm on the thigh. Hold for 1–3 seconds. Slowly return to starting position. Repeat on the opposite arm.

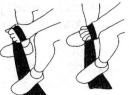

To Reduce Spinal Arthritis

Spinal arthritis problems may be the result of poor spinal alignment or posture, improper body mechanics (sitting incorrectly at a desk, poor sleeping position, lifting, twisting, or bending incorrectly), repetitive movements, or simply being out of shape. The following exercises were designed to correct problems that are associated with back pain.

Back Stretch

Position   Sit at the edge of a chair, with your feet apart and your knees and ankles aligned. Make sure the chair is stable.

Movement   Reach both hands toward the floor, relaxing your head and neck. Hold for 10–30 seconds.

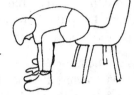

Goal   To place your palms on the floor. (This may not happen for a few days, weeks, or even months, so don't be discouraged and don't try to push beyond your physical limits.)

Calf, Hip, and Thigh Stretches

Position   Stand by a chair or a counter for support. Your feet should be shoulder-width apart, with one leg back and one leg forward. Stand tall, with your shoulders back and abdominals in. Check that your hips are square, your toes are pointing forward, and the forward knee is aligned with the ankle.

Movement for the calf stretch   Tuck the buttocks under, and straighten the knee that's behind you. Hold for 20–30 seconds. Repeat with the other leg.

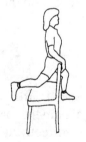

Movement for the hip stretch   Place the knee on a chair (knee behind hip), and lean the hip forward. Hold for 20–30 seconds. Repeat with the other leg.

Movement for the thigh stretch   Grab the back foot and draw it toward the buttocks. Hold for 20–30 seconds. Repeat with the other leg.

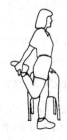

Modification   Try this if you have trouble with the standard stretch: Hold onto a counter or chair for support. Place another chair behind you. Place one knee on the back chair and lean slightly forward until you feel a stretch.

Goals To keep the knee behind the hip. To squeeze your buttocks and pull your hip forward.

Seated Thigh Stretch

Note This is a progressive stretch. Start with stage 1 until you no longer feel a stretch, then move into stage 2, and so on.

Position Sit on the edge of a chair. One leg is bent at 90 degrees (knee right above ankle), and the other leg is straight out with the toe toward the ceiling. (Do not lock your knee.)

Movement for stage 1 Place both hands on the bent leg, and lean your chest toward the bent knee. Hold for 20–30 seconds. Repeat on the other side.

Movement for stage 2 Move both hands toward the floor, straddling your bent leg. Hold for 20–30 seconds. Repeat on the other side.

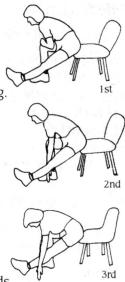

1st

2nd

Movement for stage 3 Straddling the straight leg, place hands on the floor. Hold for 20–30 seconds. Repeat on the other side.

To advance When you are comfortable with the third stage, try it with your toes rotated in, and then with them rotated out. Hold each position for 20–30 seconds.

3rd

Modification Stand by a counter or chair for support, chest out and shoulder blades squeezing together. Place the heel of one foot on a stool, and push your tailbone backward. The supporting knee remains slightly bent. Hold for 15–20 seconds. Repeat on the other side.

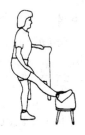

Abdominal Contraction with Diaphragmatic Breathing

Position Either lying with knees bent or sitting with back straight.

Movement Pull your abdominals in toward your 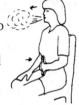 spine as you breathe out. Allow the abdominals to relax, or pouch out, as you breathe in. Do 15–25 repetitions. If you are doing this correctly, you will feel pressure in your lower back as you exhale.

Goal To retrain the body to breathe correctly.

Side Stretch

Position Sit tall with both buttocks on a chair.

Movement Reach your right arm up over your 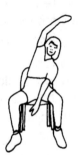 head while bending to the left and keeping your buttocks squarely on the chair. Reach up, over, and back as you pull your abdominals in. Do not let your right shoulder drop forward. Drop your left shoulder toward the floor. Hold for 15 seconds. Repeat on the other side.

Back and Side Stretch

Position Sit on the edge of a chair, feet together and knees aligned with ankles.

Movement Twist to one side, and hang both arms toward the floor (on the same side). Hold for 15–20 seconds. Repeat on the other side.

Modification If you can't perform a full twist, begin by straddling your leg; gradually work toward a twist by walking your hands around.

Goals To place your hands on the floor and then reach your elbow toward your ear. To keep your shoulders parallel to the floor.

Seated/Lying Hip and Buttock Stretch

Position   Sit tall with both buttocks on the chair. Place one ankle on the opposite thigh.

Movement   Apply pressure to the crossed thigh. Hold for 15 seconds. Move the opposite shoulder toward the crossed knee as you hug the knee into your chest and toward the opposite shoulder. Hold for 15 seconds. Straighten your back, and hold for 5 seconds. Repeat on the other side.

Goals   To keep your buttocks squarely on the chair. To sit tall with your back straight.

Modification   If this stretch is too difficult for you, it can also be done lying on the floor.

Position   Lie on your back with your knees bent. Place your ankle on the opposite knee.

Movement   Push your knee out by applying pressure to the crossed thigh. Hold for 15–30 seconds. Lift your shoulders off the floor, and hug the bent leg. Pull your foot off the floor as you move your knee toward your head (keep the thigh pressed out). Hold for 15 seconds. Repeat on the other side.

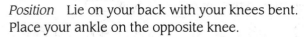

Pelvic Tilt

Position   Lie on the floor or another hard surface, feet flat and knees bent. Place your arms on the floor.

Movement   Breathe by pulling in your abdominal muscles (see page 152). Use your back muscles to flatten the lower back into the floor. Hold for 5 seconds, then relax. Do 25 repetitions.

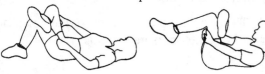

Goal   To relax your buttocks and upper torso so that you only contract the lower trunk muscles.

Lower Trunk Rotation

Position   Lie on the floor or another hard surface, knees bent and shoulders flat against the floor.

Movement for stage 1   Move both knees to one side, and hold for 15 seconds. Come back to center, then move both knees to the opposite side and hold for 15 seconds.

Movement for stage 2   Lift your knees toward your chest, turn to one side, and hold for 15 seconds. Come back to center, then turn to the opposite side and hold.

1st

To advance   Apply pressure to the top knee, using the hand closest to your rotated knees. This will increase the stretch.

2nd

Hint   It's important to keep both shoulders on the floor.

To advance

Goal   To have your bent legs relaxed against the floor without the opposite shoulder rising.

Abdominal Crunches

Position   Lie on the floor or another hard surface, feet flat and knees bent.

Movement   With your hands at your sides, perform the pelvic tilt and exhale (see page 153) as you lift your head and shoulders off the floor. Move your hands toward your ankles as you lift. Hold for 1–2 seconds, then release briefly as you relax and inhale. Build up to 2 sets of 25.

Hint   Your neck and head should be in a rigid position. Pretend to be holding an apple between your chin and chest while lifting.

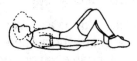

Note   This is a small movement. Your shoulders should not lift more than 4–7 inches off the floor. Also, your neck should not feel strained; be sure your abdominal muscles are doing the work.

Passive Trunk Extension

Position   Lie on your abdomen, arms bent at your sides.

Movement   Using your arms, slowly lift your torso. Support the torso with your elbows as you hold for 20–40 seconds.

Note   You should feel your abdominal muscles stretching but should not feel strain in your low back. If you experience any pain, discontinue this exercise immediately.

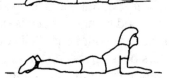

90° Wall Slides

Position   Stand with your back against a wall; your feet should be 1–2 feet from the wall. Press your head and shoulders firmly against the wall, so that your upper body is correctly aligned. Check the alignment of your legs and feet, too; when you slide down the wall, your knees and ankles should be parallel.

Movement   Slide down the wall (moving toward a sitting position but going only as far as you can tolerate), and then perform a strong pelvic tilt (see page 153). Hold for 15 seconds. Slide back up the wall. Repeat 10 times. (If your legs begin to shake, go only half as far down as you went at first.)

Hint Keep your tailbone on the wall as you flatten your back.

Note This is a fundamentally important exercise in order to control the pelvis and trunk. It will take a few attempts before you are able to perform this correctly. Follow this exercise with the back stretch and the calf, hip, and thigh stretches (pages 150 and 152).

Goals To maintain the pelvic tilt and correct posture, feeling this in your lower abdomen. To have your buttocks and knees on the same plane. To keep your head, shoulders, spine, and buttocks pressed firmly against the wall.

Side Bend

Position Stand tall, knees slightly bent and feet about shoulder-width apart for good balance. Place your left hand on top of your head. Pull your shoulders back, and keep your lower body stationary. Look straight ahead.

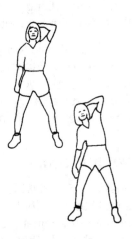

Movement Bend to the right until you feel a stretch along your left side. Pull your abdominals in, and forcefully exhale as you lift back to center. Do 10 repetitions.

Note Follow this exercise with the abdominal contractions and the side stretch (page 152).

Wide Knee Squats

Position Your feet should be more than shoulder-width apart, with your toes and knees pointed at a 45-degree angle to your body and your arms extended forward for balance.

Movement Move your body weight onto your heels as you sit back and down (you bend at the hip *and* the knees). Keep your back straight. As you lift, pull your abdominal muscles in and exhale.

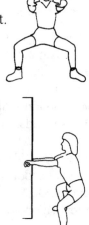

Modification If you can't do this exercise because of instability, use a counter or door handle for balance. Try the freestanding squat again in 3 weeks.

Hint If this squat causes discomfort, do the knee extensions and knee curls (page 158) for 3–6 weeks before trying squats again. These movements will strengthen your legs and help you to perform the wide-knee squat.

Note Follow the wide-knee squats with the back stretch and the calf, hip, and thigh stretches (pages 149 and 150).

Hip Wide Squats

Position Feet are hip-width apart, toes and knees pointing forward and arms extended forward for balance.

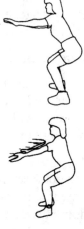

Movement Move your body weight onto your heels as you sit back and down (you bend at the hip *and* the knees). Keep your back straight. As you lift, pull your abdominals in and exhale.

Modification If you can't do this exercise because of instability, use a counter or door handle for balance. Try the freestanding squat again in 3 weeks.

Knee Extensions

Position for stage 1   Sit on a chair with your back straight.

Movement for stage 1   Lift your left foot approximately 1 inch off the floor, then extend the left leg until the knee is straight. (As you straighten your leg, pull your abdominals in and exhale.) Hold for 3–5 seconds, then slowly bend your knee to return to the starting position, with your foot still 1 inch off the floor. Do not rest your foot on the floor between repetitions. Do 10–25 repetitions. Repeat the exercise on your right side.

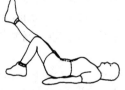

Position for stage 2   Lie on your back with your legs together and knees bent. Make certain your knees stay together.

Movement for stage 2   Straighten your left leg as you pull in your abdominals and exhale. Bend your left leg to return to the starting position, but do not rest your foot on the floor. Do 10–25 repetitions. Repeat the exercise on your right side.

Note   Follow the knee extensions with the calf, hip, and thigh stretches (page 150).

Knee Curls

Position   Lean your elbows on a counter or the back of a chair, and tighten your abdominal muscles. Keep your knees parallel, with one knee slightly behind the other. The supporting (forward) knee is slightly bent.

Movement   Lift your back foot up toward the buttocks, and hold for 1–2 seconds. Lower your foot, but do not rest it on the floor between repetitions. Do 10–25 repetitions. Repeat on the other side.

Note Follow this exercise with the seated thigh stretch (page 151).

TO REDUCE
CERVICAL SPINE ARTHRITIS

Cervical spine arthritis can result from acute injuries or trauma (falls, whiplash) or from improper body mechanics or improper position (poor sleeping posture, poor spinal alignment). And neck pain can contribute to headache pain.

Whatever the basis for your neck pain, it can typically be reduced with a flexibility, strengthening, and proper spinal alignment exercise program. By increasing the strength of the supporting structures of the spine (muscles, tendons, ligaments, discs, vertebrae), the mechanical loads and stressors are taken off the head and neck, thereby possibly resulting in reduced pain. Exercise activity can also produce proper spinal alignment of the neck, which can lead to marked reduction in neck pain and prevention of future injury. A strong neck is a healthy neck, and with this, one can resist the forces of injury.

Shoulder Shrugs

Position Stand with arms relaxed at your sides.

Movement Lift shoulders to ears and circle back and down. Repeat 10 times.

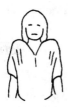

Note Squeeze shoulder blades together on the rotation backward. At no time should shoulder rotate forward.

Flexion and Extension

Position Stand with arms relaxed at your sides.

Movement Move chin to chest and push shoulders down. As you elevate chin to ceiling, shrug shoulders and hold for 1–2 seconds to enhance the stretch in extended position, push chin up. Repeat 10 times in each direction.

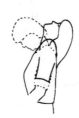

Note This can also be used as a stretch. Hold each position for 10–20 seconds.

Lateral Flexion

Position Stand with arms relaxed at your sides. Shoulders should be relaxed and down.

Movement Lift right ear to ceiling and left ear to shoulder. Hold for 1–2 seconds, then move back to center. Repeat on other side.

Note This can also be used as a stretch. Hold each position for 10–20 seconds.

Neck Rotation

Position Stand with arms relaxed at your sides.

Movement Rotate chin and ear to side, hold 1–2 seconds, then look down at shoulder. Move back to center. Rotate in the opposite direction.

Note This can also be used as a stretch. Hold each position for 10–20 seconds.

Neck Retraction

Position Stand with your arms relaxed at your sides.

Movement Squeeze shoulder blades together. Pull head straight back keeping jaw and eyes level. Hold for 5–10 seconds and relax. Repeat 10 times. Try to focus on proper posture during retraction.

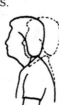

Note Do not drop or lift chin.

Chest and Shoulder Stretch

Position   Stand with your arms relaxed at your sides.

Movement   Squeeze shoulder blades together, then clasp hands behind body and extend arms.

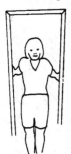

Keeping arms straight, gently lift hands and elbows toward the ceiling. Stand tall. Hold for 10–30 seconds.

Note   Hold the neck retracted while squeezing shoulder blades together.

Modification   This can also be done by placing hands on a doorway and passing torso through entrance.

Shoulder Retraction

Position   Stand with fingers touching the ears and elbows up.

Movement   Pinch shoulder blades together (as you do this, your elbows will move back). Hold for 5 seconds and release shoulder blades. Do not pull or push on the neck.

Note   Hold the neck retracted (see above) while squeezing shoulder blades together.

Modification   If it is painful to have hands behind your ears, then place hands on shoulders.

Neck Stretch

Position   Sit on a chair or stand with your arms relaxed at your sides.

Movement   Lift right ear to ceiling. Grasp right arm above wrist (in front of body) and drop shoulders as you gently pull your right

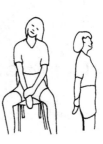

arm down. Hold for 10 seconds. Repeat with same arm behind back. Repeat to the other side.

Note   To enhance this stretch, rotate chin up and down.

Upper Back Stretch

Position for stage 1   Clasp hands together in front of body with both arms extended.

Movement for stage 1   Gently pull shoulder blades apart and drop chin to chest. Hold for 10–30 seconds.

Position for stage 2   Sit in a chair, cross arms, and grab arm rests.

Movement for stage 2   Move your chin to your chest as you open shoulder blades.

Prone Retraction

Position   Lie on the corner of a bed, face down, head and neck relaxed.

Movement   With arms bent and elbows raised, squeeze shoulder blades together, raising elbows, and hold for 5 seconds. Build up to holding for 15 seconds. Repeat 5 times.

Note   Place a pillow under your hips for support.

Repeat Upper Back Stretch (above).

Abdominal Crunches

Position   Lie on your back with knees bent and feet flat on the floor.

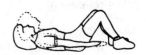

Movement   With hands at your side, lift your head and shoulders off the floor, moving hands either toward ankles or knees as you lift.

Notes   Head should be in a rigid position (pretend to have an apple between your chin and chest while lifting). Also, it is normal for the neck muscles to become fatigued.

Arm Lift

Position   Lie on the corner of a bed face down, with head and neck relaxed.

Movement   Extend arms over your head and raise arms toward the ceiling. Hold for 2–5 seconds, increasing to 15 seconds over time. Repeat 5 times.

Note   Place a pillow under your hips for support.

Repeat Chest and Shoulder Stretch (page 161) and Upper Back Stretch (page 162).

Stabilization of Shoulder Girdle

Position   Lie on the corner of a bed face down. Relax head and neck, with arms extended out to the side.

Movement   Squeeze shoulder blades together and raise both arms toward the ceiling. Hold for 5–10 seconds. Build up to holding for 20 seconds.

Note   This exercise will become easier over time. It can be advanced by holding soup cans and then weights. Reduce your hold time to 1–3 seconds.

Note   Place a pillow under your hips for support.

Repeat Upper Back Stretch (page 162).

Upper Back and Neck Stretch

Position   Stand with arms relaxed at your sides.

Movement   Tilt head to the right side and
gently grasp the left side of your head (at
ear) with your right hand, and allow gravity
to stretch the muscles. Then place left hand
behind back. Hold for 10–20 seconds.
Repeat on opposite side.

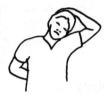

Note   Do not pull on head and neck!

Shoulder Reach

Position   Lie on your back with arms
extended toward the ceiling.

Movement   Attempt to open your shoulder
blades as you push arms straight up to the
ceiling. Keep your back against the floor and
elbows straight. Hold for 5 seconds and
build up to 15 seconds.

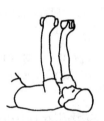

Repeat Chest and Shoulder Stretch (page 161).

Shoulder Blade Lift

Position   Stand and place left hand on left
shoulder blade, elevating elbow.

Movement   Move chin and nose to right
shoulder. Gently place right hand on top of
head and allow gravity to stretch the muscle.
Hold 10–20 seconds, repeat to the other side.

Note   Do not pull on head and neck.

Upward Row

Position   Stand tall with shoulder blades squeezing together.
Hold a towel with both hands in front of your body, palms
facing toward the body.

Movement   Leading with the elbows, lift both
hands to the chin and hold; squeeze shoulder
blades together in this position.

To advance   Once this becomes familiar,
add 1–5 pound weights, repeat 10–20 times.

Goals   At the height of the exercise, elbows should be higher
than the ears and wrists.

Repeat Neck Stretch (page 161) and Upper Back and Neck
Stretch (page 164).

───── ACTIVITIES FOR DAILY LIVING ─────

The remainder of this chapter shows you how best to perform everyday functions to keep your body properly aligned.
Good posture and proper form when walking, standing,
sleeping, lifting, and so forth will help you prevent further
pain and injury.

The standard mechanical stress load to the spine is 100
percent when standing with correct posture; we've included
here some mechanical stress percentages to give you an
idea of the stress to your body when performing certain
functions.

Walking Posture

As you begin to walk, consciously pull your head, neck, and shoulders back. Heel should strike first while pushing off with the toes of the back foot. As you step forward, lift trunk tall and pull abdominals in.

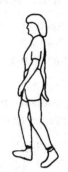

This may feel strange at first, but remember you are not used to walking or moving with correct alignment. Eventually this will feel natural.

Prolonged Standing Technique

While standing for prolonged periods of time, stagger feet shoulder-width apart and shift weight from one leg to the other. To alleviate pressure on the lower back while ironing or doing dishes, stand close to the ironing board or sink with one leg elevated 2–4 inches off the floor. Avoid leaning forward from the pelvis, back, or shoulders.

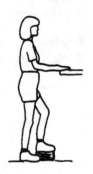

Note   Keep a soft knee, abdominals in, shoulders back, and raised sternum (breast bone). Keep your head and neck back.

Frequent One-Minute Breaks

The one-minute break is designed to enable you to change position frequently. Take time to get up and move around. Perform a few of the exercises you have learned. Use the corner stretch to help you stretch the chest and straighten your posture. Walk around your desk or office. Go to the bathroom.

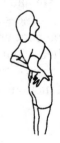

Do anything that gets you moving.

Using the Telephone

When talking on the telephone, keep your head level, with shoulders and neck back. Try not to hold the telephone with your shoulder elevated and head tilted to the side. This holds stress and tension in the upper back and neck.

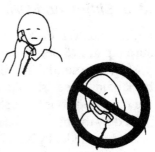

Sleeping

Improper sleeping posture increases the mechanical stress on the spine. The tightness in the soft tissues of the pelvis and legs, coupled with poor hip alignment, can be a source of discomfort along the whole spine. This can lead to neck spasm. The following rules will aid in supporting the spine and pelvis as well as reducing the mechanical stress to the spine.

- Sleep on a firm mattress to reduce tension caused by excessive curvature.

- If you sleep on your side: place a pillow in between your knees. This will reduce the mechanical stress to 75 percent.

- If you sleep on your back: place a pillow under your knees. This will reduce the mechanical stress to 5 percent. With legs extended, stress increases to 150 percent.

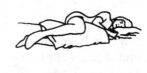

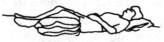

- If you sleep on your abdomen: place a pillow underneath your hips.

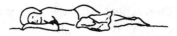

Ideal Sitting and Driving Posture

Sitting causes the greatest increase in spine pressure (up to 275 percent); therefore, proper sitting posture is essential in order to reduce chronic back pain. Knees should be slightly higher than the hips, and your back should be firmly supported by the back of the chair or seat. The chair back should ideally be on an incline and have arm rests.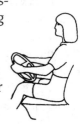

Keep head and neck retracted and abdominals in. While driving, keep both hands on the steering wheel, in the ten and two o'clock positions, for support. Be certain that you are close enough to the foot pedals so that you do not have to reach for them.

Note   Sit in correct posture. Adjust all mirrors to accommodate this posture. The mirrors will act as a reminder to correct your position when your posture fails. Also, place a rolled towel in the natural curve of your lower back to add support and to remind you to remain in correct posture.

Mechanical Stress to the Low Back:
  Sitting with proper posture: 140 percent
  Sitting with improper posture: up to 275 percent

Getting Out of Bed or Off the Couch

Using proper mechanics to get out of bed will reduce unnecessary tension on the spine. Before getting out of bed, bring knees to chest and grasp legs under knees. Pull into chest and raise shoulders to meet knees. Hold 10–30 seconds, release, then repeat. This will help you get ready to move. Roll onto your side and use your free arm to help push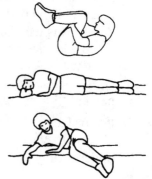

your torso up while you simultaneously swing your feet and legs off the bed or couch. This will leave you in a seated position.

Standing and Sitting

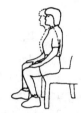

Using the proper technique to stand and/or sit will strengthen the legs and reduce discomfort and stress on the vertebrae.

To stand: Move to the edge of the chair. Place feet shoulder-width apart with one foot slightly in front of the other (back foot should be placed slightly under chair). Lean forward from the hips. Lift body with your legs. Stand erect and in good posture.

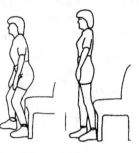

To sit: Stand tall with shoulder blades squeezing together. Back calf against the chair. Feet should be shoulder-width apart with one foot slightly in front of the other foot. Pull abdominals in, push hips back, and bend knees. Using the legs, ease back into the chair.

Getting In and Out of a Car or Confined Space

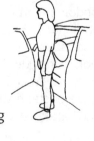

Always get in and out of a car without twisting or separating the legs. This leaves the pelvis in an unsupported position—increasing the mechanical stress on the spine. To get into a car, turn your body so that your back is facing the seat. Use proper sitting technique to sit in the car seat, then swing both legs into the car simultaneously. Getting out of the car is the exact opposite. Begin by moving both legs out of the car (using a full body turn).

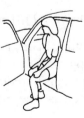

Place one foot in front of the other, lean forward from the hips, and stand erect. Keep shoulders back and chest elevated.

Half Kneeling

Move to the edge of your chair. Place one foot in front of the other with back leg under chair. With back flat and abs in tight, lean forward from the hips while pressing through the heel on your front leg, lift up and back 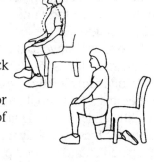 onto the chair. This technique is great for getting clothes out of the dryer, getting things out of low cabinets, and so on.

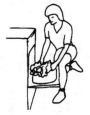

Getting Off the Floor

Half kneeling is a precursor to getting off the floor.

Roll onto all fours. Pull abdominal muscles in tight, walk hands back toward knees, and move into a kneeling position using your bent leg for support. You can now get into a chair or stand straight up using the half-kneeling technique.

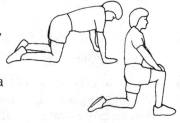

Proper Lifting and Transporting Techniques

Lifting in any position will increase the mechanical load on the spine. The mechanical advantage to lifting with proper technique is to reduce the compressive forces on the spine and increase the stability of the spine during lifting and transport.

Stand with correct posture, place feet shoulder-width apart with one foot slightly in front of the other. Pull the abs in tight and lean forward from the hips while bending the knees (squatting down). Pick up the object (using your legs to lift), tighten abs, and exhale as you slowly lift to an upright position. Keep object close to your body and in front of you as you transport item to its new location.

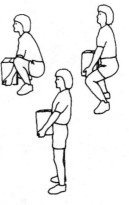

Note   Shifting the weight load to one side increases disc pressure and muscle activity on the opposite side.

Goal   Lift slowly and in a controlled manner; disc pressure increases with faster lifts and heavier loads.

Other Helpful Hints

- Lighten pocketbook and switch shoulders frequently. This will keep you from leaning and/or favoring one side.

- Avoid wearing high heels (higher than one inch above the sole of the shoe). These tend to tilt the pelvis forward and increase the curvature in the low back.

- Obesity greatly increases both the direct and indirect compressive loads on the spine by shifting center of gravity and increasing the curvature of the spine. Weight loss could reduce your pain. (See Chapter 8.)

- Stand with your arms behind your back. This will help you to keep your shoulders from rounding forward.

10

Injection Therapy
and Surgery

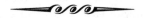

Surgery is our last option—an option we recommend only to our patients who suffer intractable pain, progressive deficits, or such severe deterioration of the joint capsule of affected arthritis joints that traditional or alternative therapies and other support therapies have no chance of succeeding without surgical assistance. Advising patients to go "under the knife" is a last resort for us. Instead, in many cases injection therapy can facilitate significant improvements.

In this chapter, we discuss injection therapy in the joints. We also talk about the role for surgery: when it should be considered and what you can hope for.

Joint Injection Therapy

You may know some people who have said that a cortisone shot in their shoulder cleared up their bursitis. Or you may have heard about individuals with terrible arthritis in the knee joint, who after one isolated cortisone injection were miraculously able to return to their full athletic and social activities, with no recurrence of pain. While these situations are certainly a possibility, we don't see them often. Instead, injecting cortisone into an inflamed joint is far more likely to serve as a short-term or intermediate solution for arthritis of that joint.

In joint injection therapy, typically the afflicted joint is numbed with a medication such as Xylocaine or Novocain (similar to the type of medicine used by dentists). When the joint feels numb, a cortisone-type material is injected directly into the joint capsule. The doctor determines the dosage of cortisone by considering the size of the joint (the larger the joint, the greater amount of cortisone) and how frequently the joints will need more injections later on.

Before receiving an injection, patients are advised to limit their activity; this limits the inflammation of the joint prior to therapy. Then, following the injection, patients are routinely instructed to rest over the next twelve to twenty-four hours, to help the effect remain localized. Ice may be recommended to reduce swelling and inflammation and any pain from the injection itself. Injection specialists who manage patients with acute and chronic pain of arthritic joints often recommend heat to the muscles and joints over the twenty-four hours following a joint injection. This can increase the blood flow and circulation, thereby improving the overall healing effect.

The pain-free period following an injection is an opportunity for the patient to begin an aggressive exercise and strengthening program, with the goal of decreasing joint inflammation and pain and minimizing the need for future injections.

Patients ask us how often they can receive injections. In the case of spinal arthritis, we typically recommend that the joint injections occur no more than three to four times per year, possibly up to six, depending on the patient's clinical condition. Certainly, weekly injections are inappropriate and would actually lead to damage and deterioration of the joint itself. The cortisone will ultimately delay healing if given in a repeated, successive fashion. But when used appropriately, cortisone injections can reduce inflammation and allow the body's natural healing forces to take over and improve the joint, bone, and cartilage as well as reduce the inflammation in the joint space itself.

Types of Injections

There are different types of cortisone injections, including short-term and longer-acting steroids. Your doctor will decide which type to use, based on your specific clinical condition, how severely inflamed the joint is, and the type of follow-up care.

Noncortisone injections have also been used on arthritis patients. In the past, doctors injected a cartilage-type material. However, recent studies do not support this type of injection. A study compared the results for three groups: people receiving cartilage-type injections, people receiving placebo (no medication), and people receiving no therapy. The cartilage and placebo groups did better than the no-therapy group; the cartilage therapy was somewhat better than the placebo therapy. When it comes to long-term management of arthritis pain, only the cortisone injection has been shown to offer any significant or long-term benefit.

Possible Risks

Injections frequently are effective. However, occasionally the steroid injections will irritate the joint capsule and can inflame the cartilage and the fluid in the joint space. If this happens, pain will increase, and the "cure" is worse than the disease. In such a case, a joint aspiration is usually sufficient. A joint aspiration involves the removal of joint fluid, which also extracts the inflammatory cortisone agent and enables the joint to recover.

Keep in mind that there is always a risk for infection any time the skin surface is injected. While this risk is considered minimal, it does exist, and the more injections you need, the higher the risk for infection.

Surgery

Surgery may be the answer for you if you've tried most of the traditional and alternative therapies outlined in this book and if you've lost weight, exercised, and followed your physician's and your exercise physiologist's instructions—but you still have severe pain. Assuming that plain x-rays reveal that your joints are continuing to degenerate, especially your hip and knee joints (the large weight-bearing joints of the body), then surgery may indeed be a consideration for you.

One red flag for surgery is when patients start to lose the ability to walk. The inability to walk can be the first step in a downward spiral toward declining general health. Consequently, surgery should perhaps be considered, as its risks are outweighed by possible benefits.

Joint Replacement Therapy

Every type of joint can be replaced—including jaw, knee, spine, and finger joints. A great deal has been written on knee surgery and hip surgery especially, and at most hospitals, the positive outcome rate is very high. When major joints are replaced, they are expected to last ten to fifteen years, depending on the patient's general health and fitness and how well the patient works to combat arthritis after surgery. Remember, joint surgery can alleviate the acute aggravation of a chronic illness—but it is not a cure. The underlying chronic illness is still there and will progress if the patient does not participate in an active exercise regimen and follow the therapeutic recommendations offered by the physician.

When we started out in our medical training, patients who had to undergo total hip replacement would often be in the hospital for weeks. Now many patients are home in three to five days. Of course, not all patients can be discharged in a few days, but certainly the sooner patients can leave the hospital, the less likely they will suffer in-hospital complications or progressive muscle weakness from lying in bed.

Techniques have improved to the point that joint repair surgery is a hard science as well as a medical art in this day and age. New techniques and materials are constantly being developed for surgical joint replacement. Recent advancements include new types of artificial "discs" for the spine, sterilized sea corral instead of bone being used to stabilize joints and the spine, and new mechanical joints that allow for greater function and range of motion.

Make sure you ask your doctor to discuss *all* the options with you!

Outpatient Surgery

Knee joint surgeries can often be done on an outpatient basis, particularly arthroscopic surgery. For an arthroscopy, the surgeon uses a small microscope to perform the surgery. The surgeon looks through a microscope, which has a special surgical tool attached, to find the problem. The surgeon monitors the surgery on a video screen, which gives a detailed, enlarged view of the surgery-in-progress. Arthroscopy leads to tiny and unnoticeable surgical puncture spots rather than the large "railroad track" surgical scars that were common just years ago. Also, using a surgical microscope to see and fix the problem, rather than actually opening up the knee joint, means less inflamation of the joint capsule and less blood flow to the area. Thus, the patient can usually expect a quicker repair of the cartilage, disc, and joint than in the past and can also enjoy a faster recovery. Often the patient is left with only two small bandages for all of the work that was done!

Sometimes it is not the cartilage that is degenerating but the bony surfaces of the joint. Under direct visualization, these bone surfaces can be "scraped down," which can lead to an improved range of motion and decreased joint inflammation. It will also reduce those annoying "click" or "pop" sounds the knee joint can make, which are so common in our patients.

We stress to all our patients that surgery should not be entered into lightly. There is still the risk associated with general anesthesia, and these patients are often considered high-risk to start with. There is always a risk for infection or a hospital-based complication.

Case Study: Tom

Tom was a patient with severe degeneration of the hip joint. He was in constant agony, but because of his age (forty-three years), he was told that he couldn't have surgery because he was too young. He was unable to work or support his family. Tom continued to suffer from severe pain, and he asked for and received narcotic tablets, but he always had distressing side effects from the narcotics. Tom decided that he did not want to live on pain pills—but what could he do?

Then things got worse, and Tom began to develop spine pain and spinal arthritis. His blood pressure went up, too. He found another doctor, who also explained the limitations of early hip replacement surgery, yet he was willing to operate if Tom was sure he wanted to proceed. He was.

Within thirty-six hours of the postoperative phase, Tom discontinued all narcotic medications. Although he had postoperative pain, he considered it "nothing compared to my joint pain." Within a few weeks, Tom was able to rehabilitate his joint, strengthen his legs, and increase the flexibility and function of his low back spine. He also enjoyed a near resolution of his spinal arthritis.

Tom still has hip joint discomfort today, but he is now able to walk and he no longer needs his wheelchair or even his crutches. While he has not returned to a vigorous type of work, he has been able to work at a desk job, and he has been able to financially provide for his family. His self-esteem has greatly improved. Tom is well on his way to emotional and physical recovery.

Will he need this surgery again, later in life? Probably. Tom knows that he may again need joint replacement surgery in seven, ten, or fifteen years. For Tom, it was worth it.

11

The Mind-Body Connection

We've talked about the role that genetics, your diet, weight, and other elements can play if and when arthritis becomes a problem for you. This chapter centers on the mind-body connection, which is the interaction between what and how you think and how you feel.

Mood and Illness

We know that if you are in a bad or angry mood, you are more prone to illness. We also know that if you are ill, you are more likely to be distressed or even depressed. In fact, depression is a common and predictable consequence of chronic painful states—and arthritis is certainly a chronic painful state.

Many other aspects of a chronically painful condition can contribute to a patient's emotional condition. Often, individuals with chronic pain have trouble sleeping, and this is a significant risk for depression. (Sleep difficulties are discussed in

Chapters 4, 5, and 8.) Another key factor for people with (and without) chronic pain is self-image. If people cannot fulfill the roles in life they find important, whether as spouses, workers, parents, or in other roles, then there is a loss of self-esteem and decrease in self-worth. People may feel alienated from friends and family.

This can be especially true if there is no visible sign of recent trauma. You look normal, and people expect you to act normal. Maybe you look so normal that you get dirty looks when you park in the "handicapped" spaces. So you suffer through feelings of helplessness, frustration, and anger, as well as the direct physical problems caused by arthritis.

Some studies indicate that the depression resulting from chronic pain is actually a worse problem than the chronic pain condition alone. While we are not sure about this, we do know that a connection does exist. However difficult the depression may be, it's clear that there is a link between chronic pain and suffering and depression, and this can lead to a downward spiral of additional pain. Don't let this happen to you! Follow the suggestions in this book to prevent this downward spiral or to break out of it if you have already been sucked in.

How Emotions Affect the Body

It's not easy to walk around with a happy face when you're hurting. But there has been a great deal of recent scientific and alternative health information suggesting that a patient's mental well-being can and does affect physical well-being too. This concept is often referred to as psychoneuroimmunology.

We are all familiar with people who are considered low in resistance. If anything is going around, you can be sure they'll come down with it. These individuals are also less likely to be cheerful, are less likely to have a positive outlook, and are more likely to have a higher rating of pain (a higher subjective complaint). They are in a negative downward spiral.

How does it work? Simply put, a person's emotional outlook, energy, stamina, and mood can trigger chemical changes in the brain that affect the immune system. This seems to occur via chemical and hormonal pathways in the brain. The pituitary is a small gland that controls the flow of hormones in the body and affects endocrinologic (hormone) functions. Such chemicals include thyroid hormones, adrenaline, and production of female/male sex hormones.

When the body is stressed and patients are in poor health, an apparent breakdown occurs in the production of certain stress chemicals. This then triggers a feedback mechanism, leading to changes in the hormone messengers of the brain. To put it simply, stress leads to a change in the immune system.

The change in the immune system then leads to a breakdown in health, which leads to additional changes in the brain chemicals. The brain chemicals then affect the hormone levels in a negative fashion, which ultimately have a negative outcome on the immune system, which likewise affects the brain chemicals negatively, and so forth.

The sympathetic nervous system plays a role in the regulation and feedback of the endocrine, hormone, and neurotransmitter system of the brain. For example, adrenaline seems to interact with the activity of immune cells, with increased adrenaline levels decreasing immune cell function. This can ultimately lead to altered immune responses.

There have been many laboratory studies showing how a reduction in the fight-or-flight system (adrenaline or sympathetic system) in animals can also reduce the immune response and antibody (the body's protective immune chemicals) production to various types of illness. With this reduced response to illness, that illness can take hold in the body, spread, and lead to an infection and a recognized clinical syndrome.

Not only your true clinical condition but also your perception of your condition modulates and adjusts the production of various chemical messengers in your brain and body. Studies have demonstrated that patients with chronic illness seem to "suffer more" than would seem to be indicated from their illness; they are also reported to have lower feelings of well-being.

Let's return to the simple analogy of the leaky faucet, which we introduced in Chapter 4. When you hear a leaky faucet dripping water, the first day or week may not be too bad, but after some time, it becomes unpleasant. Over a longer period of time, it becomes unbearable agony and you can't get it out of your mind. Your kingdom to anyone who fixes that faucet! Clearly, the individual drip in the leaky faucet has not changed; the change is a lower pain threshold. This is the difference between pain and suffering.

You may also be caught up in a conditioned response, a reaction of your feelings and the subsequent sensation of illness to produce certain neurotransmitter chemicals. These chemicals regulate or decrease your immune response. They then lead to more sickness and more unhappy opportunities for additional infection or poor health. In studies of animals undergoing stressful, painful conditions, it has been proven that stressful conditions can have adverse effects on the immune system; for most of us, this is intuitively obvious.

One theory to explain this phenomenon is that stress increases the production of adrenaline as well as cortisone and therefore the immune system does not work as well. With the help of your physician and your own active efforts, you can break out of this system.

Treating the Total Patient

An important principle for a good doctor is to treat the patient, not the illness. The goal is to restore homeostasis, or a balance of all the body's natural systems. If arthritis is causing pain, the pain is causing stress, and the stress is causing stress chemicals to block the immune system, then this pathway must be interrupted. This can be done by blocking the pain, alleviating the stress, or increasing the immune response.

Treating the inflamed joints alone is not enough. In a recent nursing health magazine, groups of women with chronic illness were interviewed and evaluated. Women with positive outlooks, positive social experiences, and improved social networks had a higher rating of psychosocial well-being, independent of their organic or physical problems. Some of the women with good attitudes had the same serious illness as others who were not coping well with it at all.

Another study on arthritis, the perception of arthritis, and quality of life revealed that individuals who had improved coping mechanisms also experienced lower perceptions of pain, improved perceptions of self-worth, and reduced rating of their overall pain or suffering.

An article in the summer 1996 issue of *The Journal of Health Care Marketing* reviewed the roles of emotions in health care satisfaction. A doctor's ability to understand a patient's emotions was considered to be a critical aspect in determining whether or not patients would be successful with their health care outcome.

Part of this process lay in determining a patient's description of "successful outcome." Reduction of pain was important, but also significant to a patient's rating of health care satisfaction were improvements in self-image, general wellness, and energy and stamina.

The Physician's Role

As we see it, a physician can intervene anywhere along this pathway of pain, fatigue, stress, depression, and inactivity. Doctors can help to decrease depression and increase the motivation of patients with chronic arthritis pain.

Traditional psychiatrists treating depression have known for a long time that many medications are very effective for depression. A broad variety of antidepressants fall into several classes: tricyclic antidepressants, selective serotonin reuptake inhibitors, and mixed reuptake inhibitors. Basically what this means is that certain antidepressants affect certain chemical messengers of the brain.

In our own practice, clearly we believe the patients should be active participants when it comes to intervening with their pain. (See Chapter 5 for our discussion on multiple management techniques and alternative therapies.) Here are some simple guidelines that we take to intervene with our patients, addressing the total patient and not just their arthritis illness.

First, we obtain a total history, not one that deals solely with the medical illness. We also obtain information from the patient and other family members regarding quality of life and pain history. This provides us with a comprehensive outline of how this painful condition is impacting not only the patient's health but also the person's life. Next, we perform a physical examination, using the necessary laboratory and diagnostic testing. (See Chapter 3 outlining the doctor visit.)

Then we move on to therapeutic intervention. This includes outlining an exercise regimen (our staff members see us demonstrating various stretching, strengthening, and range of motion exercises to our patients). Often patients will state that they can't do it, because "it hurts too much." We stress once again the slow and steady course: start low, go slow.

We believe strongly in proper body mechanics and have outlined proper mechanisms for patients to perform routine daily activities. Surprisingly, patients can go from physician visit to physician visit or even therapy visit to therapy visit, all without ever learning how to sit, how to stand, how to get in and out of a car, how to bend over, or how to get up from the floor. Not only do we have our therapists teach these simple activities of daily life (see pages 165 to 171), but we also offer a video, "Spinal Tips" (1-800-844-7880), which demonstrates these techniques. These little intervention activities can go a long way in reducing pain and flare-ups.

The Patient's Role

In helping our patients, we correct life activities such as nutrition, diet, and sleep cycle, and we explain how certain activities can lead to additional stress. Patients at some level know that certain patterns in their job, relationships, home life, or extracurricular activities are probably not good for them, yet some continue to follow the same pattern.

As we have seen, stress can have a negative impact on the immune system, which ultimately can lead to additional inflammatory processes of the already damaged arthritic joints; certainly the opposite must be true. A peaceful, relaxed work environment, home environment, and social environment would certainly go a long way in reducing additional painful flare-ups and in initiating a curative process.

Proper Diet   We are not nutritionists, but we do know that patients need to be well aware of the role of diet as well as the role of toxins in the body. It's important to make appropriate life choices to empower you to not only feel well but to ultimately be well. (For more information on diet, see Chapter 8.)

Weight Loss   If you have arthritis and need to lose weight, it's very important to start now. Maybe you'll need to join an fitness center that takes into account your problem. Maybe you'll need weight loss medication, such as Redux (see page 119 for further information). You may also need to join a club or group that is oriented to weight loss, although we recommend organizations with low fees or no fees (such as Overeaters Anonymous).

You also need to consult with your physician—this is imperative. Patients who are over their ideal body weight should certainly seek medical attention, nutritional guidance, and exercise assistance to learn to reduce their body weight to their target goal. Working with your doctor on a plan to drop those pounds, you can reduce your risk for additional medical problems and reduce your arthritis pain.

Psychiatric Help   You don't have to be "crazy" to see a psychiatrist; most of the patients these medical doctors see are normal people facing difficult problems. Sometimes people need a little extra help, and a psychiatrist can provide good advice and assistance.

Forget those images of lying on a soft leather couch and saying whatever comes into your head, day after day. That's psychoanalysis, and this Woody Allen kind of therapy has been discredited today. The overwhelming majority of psychiatrists concentrate on helping their patients work on problem-solving over the short term, and they may see a person once a week or monthly or even four times a year.

Helpful listening can be beneficial for a patient who is having difficulty coping with pain and illness; it can help the patient understand this normal process of chronic pain, and it can often be the first step in overcoming this co-morbid condition.

Once again, we stress that patients need to maintain a positive outlook as much as possible, particularly with regard to their chronic pain. This is very important. Many articles have outlined the positive benefits of a positive outlook. Although it is natural to be upset when you don't feel well, it's very important to do your best to maintain a positive mental attitude. If you don't, it's almost like taking one step toward more pain. An upbeat attitude—sometimes in combination with pain medication, antidepressants, other treatments, and exercise—can move you away from that pain demon and closer and closer to wellness.

12

The Future Looks Bright

In this chapter, we focus on new technologies and concepts in health care that will be affecting people with arthritis very soon. In fact, some new breakthroughs already appear to be creating a cure, such as cloning therapy and genetic therapy. As a result, this is a very exciting time for health care practitioners. Every day we are learning more and more about the body, the role of behavior and pain, and new remedies; and we are coming closer to alleviating your pain.

Bloodless Surgery

As we discuss in Chapter 10, surgery should only be a last resort. However, in the future, even surgery may not be surgery as we know it now. Already, "bloodless surgery" enables surgeons to excise various tumors and nervous system lesions with a gamma radiation laser knife. By using computer technology, surgeons can three-dimensionally identify the location of the tumor and, with the appropriate depth of radiation, perform a surgical laser therapy of the tumor, with no additional invasion of the body.

We have had patients who have benefited from this exciting new technology. It's amazing to see patients who once had serious spinal cord or brain tumors, now in full recovery of their tumor condition, with no surgical marks on their bodies. Even an experienced physician would never know that surgery had been performed. In addition, the surgery was accurate, bloodless, and relatively painless, and it produced a cure.

We believe that over the next several years, this type of technology will expand, not only to the nervous system but also into the musculoskeletal system in general and to inflamed and damaged joint capsules in particular. As a result, bloodless surgery holds great promise for individuals suffering from arthritis who need surgery for their severe, chronic, and intractable arthritis pain.

Cold Laser Treatment

Along the same lines as bloodless surgery, laser therapy now exists and is being used for the treatment of nerve and muscle pain. Starting in 1997, this technology is making its way into mainstream therapy approaches to muscle, ligament, and joint pains. There are two types of laser treatments for pain: hot and cold. The hot laser, which heats and burns, is often used in surgery; it is not useful in current arthritis care.

The cold laser is a deep-penetrating laser. A number of research protocols are currently underway to explain the benefits of the cold laser. Clearly it is considered safe and has been classified as a "nonsignificant health risk device," but it has not yet been approved by the FDA. Neurologists, rheumatologists, and chiropractic physicians all know about this therapy, which has been effective in veterinarian care for some time. It is just now becoming available for human patients.

The concept behind the cold laser is that the wave lengths it generates are able to penetrate soft tissue. In this way, the laser gets into the muscle ligament or inflamed joint and may stimulate the blood flow around the inflamed area. (Some individuals call this photo biostimulation.)

A neurologist in New York has used this method to treat patients successfully. He has measured nerve conduction across the wrist joint before and after treatment. After several sessions, he has found that these nerve conduction cases have all returned to normal. There is no pain, and patients have stated that the very first session reduced some of their discomfort. This treatment seems more effective for the smaller joints, such as the fingers, wrists, elbows, and knees. The hip joints and shoulder joints seem to be less improved following a trial of therapy.

This therapy is in its infancy, and we are certain that over the next three to five years we will see the advent of a variety of probes, techniques, and ancillary care using the cold laser. These treatments will enable doctors to reduce joint swelling, inflammation, and ultimately pain.

Nutritional Breakthroughs

In Chapter 8, we discuss nutrition and diet and the effect of diet on behavior, outlook, mood, alertness, speed of thought, and pain sensitivity. We are certain that new diet combinations will be found to benefit patients with arthritis. This rapidly expanding field of medicine is called nutritional neuropharmacology. We have no doubt that the combination of diet, relaxation therapy, EEG evaluation, and biofeedback will play a significant role in a long-term solution to arthritis pain.

Cloning Breakthroughs

In Chapter 10 on surgery, we discuss cartilage injections. In the past, these injections were found to be no more beneficial than placebo injections. However, new therapies are on the horizon. At Beth Israel Hospital in New York, for example, cartilage can now be partially removed from the inflamed joint, cloned in the laboratory, and reinjected into the body! This cloning cartilage treatment will ultimately help to reform new cartilage.

While this treatment is very expensive today, imagine the implications. For an inflamed thumb, finger, wrist, or elbow joint (even a hip or knee joint), the physician could remove a piece of that inflamed joint, culture it in a dish, clone the cartilage, inject it back in, and voila! A new joint is born.

The technology is nearly here now and awaits only two factors: refinement of the technique and a reduction in price. Few patients can afford a $35,000 procedure. But if the technique becomes cost-effective (and it will), this combined with proper fitness and nutrition will be the cure of the future.

Gene Therapy

Looking to the future, we need to address two high-tech and scientifically ingenious approaches to arthritis care. One is gene therapy; the other is nanobiotechnology (see the next section). The goal is to alleviate the degenerative and inflammatory process of arthritis and other immune diseases affecting the joints.

The future is here now: on July 17, 1996, a sixty-eight-year-old woman became the very first patient at the University of Pittsburgh Medical Center in Pittsburgh, Pennsylvania, to receive gene therapy for arthritis. Simply put, doctors modified the patient's own cells. The cells were tagged with a special gene that blocks both inflammation and erosion of the joint. Her modified cells were then injected back into the knuckles of one hand. The procedure was a success. Her injected joints had no new inflammation or further degeneration.

By tagging the patient's cells with this immune-blocking agent, the patient's joint will not see cartilage and breakdown products as foreign substances, and consequently the patient's body will not attack these joints. This research is an exciting new approach to arthritis joint therapy, with more work to be done. The goal is complete relief of arthritis. If a physician can completely reduce pain and inflammation in the joint, hopefully on a permanent basis, then we have a cure.

Nanobiotechnology

An even more wide-thinking approach to health care is the concept of nanobiotechnology. This large scientific word simply refers to the science of breaking objects down into their basic molecular atoms and structure and then building them back up in a disease-free fashion. In this way, an atomic repair machine could be placed in the body to remove inflammation and then rebuild the human "site."

The bad news is that nanobiotechnology is decades away (or longer). However, with the rapid expansion of science and technology, this approach will ultimately become available for treating not only arthritis but also other degenerative and inflammatory disease processes. Imagine a nanobiotechnology machine that could be injected to clean out arteries, keeping the elastic tissue safe and sound while cleaning up plaque. Think about it: that extra helping of ice cream would be okay—if there were no risk of gaining weight!

The future is tremendously exciting to think about, and we are extremely optimistic that breakthroughs will enable us to help our patients. At the same time, we continue to be convinced that a healthful lifestyle, exercise, good nutrition, and proper body mechanics will ultimately be the cure for arthritis and for joint pain. Nevertheless, as long as science

Conclusion

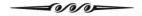

Now you know all about arthritis—or at least as much as many well-educated patients and some not-so-educated physicians know. You know that there is more than one way to approach this chronic and at times disabling and debilitating illness. And although we do not have a "cure," there are many *solutions*. We look at each and every therapy as a piece of the puzzle. When you fit the pieces that apply to your own individual situation, you can approach your illness with a sense of optimism and confidence, realizing that you can find your own arthritis solution.

As mentioned in the preface, Marie did well by combining various cure treatments including magnets, weight loss, and an exercise regimen. Two more examples here will help illustrate how other arthritis sufferers have successfully reduced the burden of their arthritis condition while at the same time increasing their energy, stamina, and overall quality of life.

Bruce, age 39, is an active and successful marketing executive and board-certified lawyer. Over the past few years, he has suffered knee joint and hip pain, the result of an old basketball injury. He has also had spine surgery for a disc problem, and he has experienced joint inflammation in the bones of the low back.

Bruce came to us distraught and frustrated. He stated, "I'm always on a plane, dragging around my legal briefs; my hip is killing me, my knee is killing me, and I'm ready for another surgery." However, the one thing Bruce hadn't counted on was that there was more than one way to treat his knee and hip pain, and we discussed numerous treatment options. Bruce volunteered that he was unable to take the traditional "anti-inflammatories" as they always hurt his stomach. However, no one had ever mentioned additional treatments to him, such as natural therapy, muscle relaxants, or alternative therapies. Bruce told us fervently, "I'll do anything if I don't have to have surgery. I just want to be well."

Bruce began an exercise regimen at a fitness center. He chose the fitness center because he knew that—given his busy lifestyle—he wouldn't exercise if it were up to him. Also, to alleviate his immediate pain, we referred him for acupuncture, which worked very well.

We also prescribed a hand-held electric stimulator, which relaxed the muscle inflammation. His acupuncturist taught him to find his acupuncture points with the stimulator. Using these combined therapies, Bruce has been able to avoid surgery and is back to wheeling and dealing. In fact, the last time we saw him, he told us that his business revenues had skyrocketed because he was free to concentrate on deals instead of on his hip and knee pain.

Bruce knows that he will have to continue his exercise, stretching, and acupressure therapy. But for Bruce this is a small price to pay.

Amy, age 38, is vice-president of her jewelry company and the mother of two very active small children. Her business requires that she attend many trade shows, flying from coast-to-coast, and she came to us because of a painful knee. She had injured her knee in a skiing accident, and it later resulted in arthritis of the knee.

A surgeon had told Amy there was no additional treatment for her knee pain—except surgery. He mentioned a few knee exercises, and that was that. Unfortunately, over the last two to three years, her knee problem had led to a hip joint inflammation caused by improper walking. In short, she was favoring her good knee. After a while, her hips and other leg were bearing more and more of the pressure. Her hip had become inflamed and degenerated.

Amy wanted a resolution to her painful problem, so she consulted pain specialists, orthopedists, family physicians, sports medicine physicians, and rheumatologists. She tried exercise, anti-inflammatories, pain pills, and muscle relaxers. Nothing helped.

When we saw Amy for a comprehensive evaluation and treatment assessment plan, we spent a few minutes talking about her lifestyle and her hectic pace. It was clear that she was a bright, assertive individual who was in charge of everything except her own health. We placed Amy in charge of her health; we taught her how to do relaxation and biofeedback, and we treated her with relaxation therapy and guided imaging.

In addition, we had her work with a psychologist briefly so she could learn some behavior modification techniques. We added supplements and nutrients to her diet, which was woefully inadequate because of her hectic and active lifestyle. Last, we began Amy on an arthritis diet, giving her lists of foods to eat and foods to avoid, so she could make intelligent choices when she was traveling.

In Amy's case, the phytonutrient therapy worked very well, giving her more energy and reducing her pain.

Her arthritis solution was not quickly evident, but after three to four months, Amy noticed a significant reduction in pain, and more impressive, a significant improvement in her function. She is now able to lift her children and walk up and down stairs without pain and aching. She was also able to resume many social and athletic activities, which she had missed sorely, especially golfing. She had thought she had given this up for good.

Amy, as with many other patients, did not have a quick fix. She still has the illness and is not "cured," but she has solved her condition to the point that she can function without pain, without pain pills, and without the side effects of traditional medical intervention.

These two examples illustrate how individuals can take control of their own arthritic condition—and that's what we hope you've learned from this book. By reviewing the information in the various chapters, you can choose what works for you and what will provide your solution. We want to hear what combination works for you, too, because this could help others.

As we mentioned in the introduction, as well as in the chapter on the doctor-patient relationship (Chapter 3), we feel very strongly that it is up to each and every patient to communicate with his or her physician. Talk about your symptoms, and make sure that what you say (and what the doctor says to you) is heard, responded to, and acted upon. We encourage our patients to be active participants in their health care and ultimate wellness, and with the tools in this book, you can do just that.

To your health!

Appendix:
Arthritis Foundation
Chapters

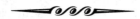

L isted below is information on Arthritis Foundation chapters. Although each chapter falls under the auspices of the national organzation, each chapter operates independently. Chapter services vary, but most offer brochures, local support groups, informational classes, forums, exercise programs, monthly newsletters, and camps for juvenile arthritis sufferers. Membership is $20 per year, but you don't have to be a member to take advantages of some services.

Alabama

Alabama Chapter
300 Vestavia Parkway, Suite
    3500
Birmingham, AL 35216
Phone: (205) 979-5700

Alaska

Alaska Unit
c/o Arthritis Foundation
1314 Spring Street, NW
Atlanta, GA 30309

Arizona

Central Arizona Chapter
777 East Missouri #119
Phoenix, AZ 85014

Southern Arizona Chapter
6464 East Grant Road
Tucson, AZ 8571
Phone: (520) 290-9090

Arkansas

Arkansas Chapter
6212 Lee Avenue
Little Rock, AR 72205
Phone: (501) 664-7242
Toll-free: (800) 482-8858
Fax: (501) 664-6588
Hours: 8:30 A.M.–4:30 P.M.
    (Central)
arkansas@aol.com

California

Northeastern California/Northern Nevada Chapter
3040 Explorer Drive
Suite 1
Sacramento, CA 95827-2729
Phone: (916) 368-5599
Toll-free: (800) 571-3456
Fax: (916) 368-5596
Hours: 8:30 A.M.–4:00 P.M.
    (Pacific)

Northern California Chapter
203 Willow Street
Suite 201
San Francisco, CA 94019
Phone: (415) 673-6882
Toll-free: (800) 464-6240
Fax: (415) 673-4101
Hours: 9:00 A.M.–5:00 P.M.
    (Pacific)

San Diego Area Chapter
9089 Clairemont Mesa Boulevard, Suite 300
Sand Diego, CA 92123-1288
Phone: (619) 492-1090
Toll-free: (800)-422-8885
Fax: (619)492-9248 or 619-492-9136
Hours: 9:00 A.M.–5:00 P.M.
    (Pacific)

Southern California Chapter
4311 Wilshire Boulevard
Suite 530
Los Angeles, CA 90010-3775
Phone: (213) 954-5750
Toll-free (800) 954-2873 (California and Nevada only)
Fax: (213) 954-5790
Hours: M-Th 8:30 A.M.–
    5:00 P.M. / F 8:30 A.M.-
    4:30 P.M. (Pacific)

Colorado

Rocky Mountain Chapter
2280 South Albion Street
Denver, CO 80222-4906
Phone: (303) 756-8622
Toll-free: (800) 475-6447
Fax: (303) 759-4349
Hours: 8:00 A.M.–4:30 P.M.
    (Mountain)

Connecticut

Connecticut Chapter
35 Cold Spring, Bldg 400
Rocky Hill, CT 06067
Phone: (203) 563-1177

Delaware

Delaware Chapter
222 Philadelphia Pike
Suite 8
Wilmington, DE 19809
Phone: (302) 764-8254
Toll-free: (800) 292-9599
Fax: (302) 764-1820
Hours: 9:00 am.–5:00 P.M.
   (Eastern)
afdc@sprynet.com

District of Columbia

*Metropolitan Washington
   Chapter*
4455 Connecticut Avenue,
   N.W.
Suite 300
Washington, DC 20008
Phone: (202) 537-6859
Fax: (202) 537-6859
Hours: 8:30 A.M.–5:00 P.M.
   (Eastern)
arthritsdc@aol.com

Florida

Florida Chapter
511 Manatee Avenue, West
Bradenton, FL 34209
Phone: (941) 795-3010
Fax: (941) 798-3659
Hours: 9:00 am.–5:00 P.M.
   (Eastern)

Georgia

Georgia Chapter
550 Pharr Road
Suite 550
Atlanta, GA 30305
Phone: (404) 237-8771
Toll-free: (800) 933-7023
   (from Georgia)
Fax: (404) 237-8153
Hours: 9:00 A.M.–5:00 P.M.
   (Eastern)

Hawaii

Hawaii Chapter
Honfed Bank Building
45-1144 Kamecharneha
   Highway
Kaneohe, HI 96744

Idaho

Utah/Idaho Chapter
448 East 400 South
Suite 103
Salt Lake City, UT 84111
Phone: (801) 536-0990
Toll-free: (800) 444-4993
   (outside the Salt Lake
   area)
Fax: (801) 536 0991
Hours: 8:30 A.M.–5:00 P.M.
   (Mountain)

Illinois

Greater Illinois Chapter
2621 N. Knoxville
Peoria, IL 61604
Phone: (309) 682-6600
Arthritis GIL@Flink, com

Greater Chicago Chapter
303 East Wacker Drive
Suite 300
Chicago, IL 60601
Phone: (312) 616-3470
Toll-free: (800) 735-0096
   (Northeast Illinois and
   Northwest Indiana only)
Fax: (312) 616-9281
Hours: 9:00 A.M.–5:00 P.M.
   (Central)
gccinfo@arthritis.org

Indiana

Indiana Chapter
8646 Guion Road
Indianapolis, IN 46268-3011

Iowa

Iowa Chapter
2600 72nd Street
Suite D
Des Moines, IA 50322-4724
Phone: (515) 278-2603
Fax: (515) 278-2603
Hours: 8:30 A.M.–4:30 P.M.
   (Central)

Kansas

Kansas Chapter
1602 East Waterman
Wichita, KS 67211
Phone: (316) 263-0116

Kentucky

Kentucky Chapter
410 W. Chestnut St., Ste. 750
Louisville, KY 40202-2325
Phone: (502) 585-1866

Louisiana

Louisiana Chapter
10473 Old Hammond Hwy.,
   Ste 201
Baton Rouge, LA 70816
Phone: (504) 929-9551

Maine

*Northern New England
   Chapter*
P.O. Box 422
257 South Union Street
Burlington, Vermont 05402
Phone: (802) 864-4988
Fax: (802) 864-5339
Hours: 8:30 A.M.–4:30 P.M.
   (Eastern)

Maryland

Maryland Chapter
1777 Reisterstown Road
Suite 150
Baltimore, MD 21108
Phone: (410) 602-0160
Toll-free: (800) 365-3811
Fax: (410) 602-0420
Hours: 8:30 A.M.–4:30 P.M.
   (Eastern)

Massachusetts

Massachusetts Chapter
29 Crafts Street
Newton, MA 02158
Phone: (617) 244-1800

Michigan

Michigan Chapter
17117 West 9 Mile Road
Suite 959
Southfield, Michigan 48075
Phone: (810) 424-9001
Fax: (810) 424-9005

Minnesota

Minnesota Chapter
830 Transfer Road
St. Paul, Minnesota
Phone: (612) 644-4108
Fax: (612) 644 4219
Hours: 8:30 A.M.–5:00 P.M.
(Central)

Missouri

Eastern Missouri Chapter
8390 Delmar Boulevard
St. Louis, MO 63124-2100
Phone: (314) 991-9333
Fax: (314) 991-4020
Hours: 8:30 A.M.–5:00 P.M.

*Western Missouri/Greater
    Kansas City Chapter*
1100 Pennsylvania Avenue,
    Suite 400
Kansas City, MO 64105-1336
Tel: (816) 842-0335
Fax: (816) 842-2847
Hours: 9:00 am.–5:00 P.M.
(Central)
arthfdn@coop.crn.org

Montana

Rocky Mountain Chapter
2280 South Albion Street
Denver, CO 80222-4906
Phone : (303) 756-8622
Toll-free: (800) 475-6447
Fax: (303) 759-4349
Hours: 8:00 A.M.–4:30 P.M.
(Mountain)

Nebraska

Nebraska Chapter
7101 Newport Avenue
Suite 304
Omaha, NE 68152
Phone: (402) 572-3040
Toll-free: (800) 642-5292
    (outside Omaha)
Fax: (402) 572-3048
Hours: 8:30 A.M.–4:30 P.M.
(Central)

Nevada

*Northeastern California/
    Norther Nevada Chapter*
3040 Explorer Drive
Suite 1
Sacramento, California
    95827-2729
Phone: (916) 368-5599
Toll-free: (800) 571-3456
Fax: (916) 368-5596
Hours: 8:30 A.M.–4:00 P.M.
(Pacific)

Southern California Chapter
Las Vegas Branch
3850 West Desert Inn Road
Suite 108
Las Vegas, NV 89102
Phone: (702) 367-1626
Fax: (702) 367-6381

New Hamphsire

Northern New England
Chapter
P.O. Box 422
257 South Union Street
Burlington, VT 05402
Phone: (802) 864-4988
Fax: (802) 864-5339
Hours: 8:30 A.M.–4:30 P.M.
(Eastern)

New Jersey

New Jersey Chapter
200 Middlesex Turnpike
Iselin, NJ 08830
Phone: (908) 283-4300
Fax: (908) 283-4633
Hours: 9:00 A.M.–5:00 P.M.
(Eastern)

New Mexico

New Mexico Chapter
124 Alvarado, S.E.
Albuquerque, NM 87108
Phone: (505) 265-1545

New York

New York Chapter
122 East 42nd Street
New York, NY 10168-1898
Phone: (212) 984-8700
Fax: (212) 878-5960

Central New York Chapter
5858 E. Molloy Road
Suite 123
Syracuse, NY 13211
Phone: (315) 455-8553
Fax: (315) 455-8714
Hours: 8:30 A.M.–4:30 P.M.
(Eastern)

Genesee Valley Chapter
2423 Monroe Avenue
Rochester, NY 14618
Phone: (716) 423-9490

Long Island Chapter
501 Walt Whitman Road
Suite 8
Melville, NY 11747
Phone: (516) 427-8272
Fax: (516) 427-3546
Hours: 8:30 A.M.–5:00 P.M.
(Eastern)
maca@pb.net

Northeastern New York
Chapter
1717 Central Avenue
Suite 105
Albany, NY 12205
Phone: (518) 456-1203
Toll-free: (800) 420-5554
Fax: (518) 869-3123
104743.2041@compuserve.com

Western New York Chapter
Tonawanda, NY 14150-9498
Phone: (716) 837-8600 (In
Buffalo)
Fax: (716) 837-8606
Hours: 9:00 am.–5:00 P.M.
(Eastern)
arthritis wyn@juno.com

North Carolina

Carolinas Chapter
7 Woodlawn Green
Suite 217
5019 Nations Crossing
Charlotte, NC 28217
Phone: (704)529-5166
Toll-free: (800)883-8806 (outside Charlotte)
Fax: (704)529-0626
Hours: 9:00 A.M.–5:00 P.M. (Eastern)

North Dakota

Dakota Chapter
c/o Arthritis Foundation
1314 Spring Street, NW
Atlanta, GA 30309
Toll-Free: (800) 872-7100

Ohio

Central Ohio Chapter
3740 Ridge Mill Drive
P.O. Box 218182
Columbus, Ohio 43221-8182
Phone: (614)876-8200
Fax: (614)876-8363
Hours: 8:30 A.M.–5:00 P.M. (Eastern)

Northeastern Ohio Chapter
23811 Chagrin Boulevard
#210
Cleveland, OH 44122-5525
Phone: (216)831-7000
Toll-free: (800)245-2275 (outside Cuyahoga County)
Fax: (216)831-1764
Hours: 9:00 A.M.–4:30 P.M. (Eastern)

Northwestern Ohio Chapter
309 North Reynolds Road
Toledo, OH 43615
Phone: (419)537-0888

Ohio River Valley
7811 Laurel Avenue
Cincinnati, OH 45243
Phone: (513)271-4703
Hours: 9:00 A.M.–5:00 P.M. (Eastern)

Oklahoma

Eastern Oklahoma Chapter
4520 S. Harvard, #100
Tulsa, OK 74135
Phone:(918)743-4526

Oklahoma Chapter
2915 Classen Boulevard, #325
Oklahoma City, OK 73106
Phone:(405)521-0066

Oregon

Oregon Chapter
4412 S. W. Barbur Blvd., Ste. 220
Portland, OR 97201
Phone: (503)222-7246

Pennsylvania

Central Pennsylvania Chapter
P.O. Box 668
17 South 19th Street
Camp Hill, PA 17011
Phone: (717)763-0900

Eastern Pennsylvania Chapter
117 South 17th Street
Architect's Building, Suite
   1905
Philadelphia, PA 19103-5097
Phone: (215)665-9200
Toll-free:(800)355-9040
Fax: (215)665-9249
Office hours: 8:30 A.M.–
   4:30 P.M. (Eastern)

Western Pennsylvania Chapter
Warner Centre–Fifth Floor
332 Fifth Avenue
Pittsburgh, PA 15222
Phone: (412)566-1645

Rhode Island

Rhode Island Chapter
37 North Blossom St.
East Providence, RI
   021914-2728
Phone: (401)434-5792

South Carolina

Carolinas Chapter
7 Woodlawn Green
Suite 217
5019 Nations Crossing
Charlotte, NC 28217
Phone: (704)529-5166
Toll-free: (800)883-8806
   (outside Charlotte)
Fax: (704)529-0626
Hours: 9:00 A.M.–5:00 P.M.
   (Eastern)

South Dakota

Dakota Chapter
c/o Arthritis Foundation
1314 Spring Street, NW
Atlanta, GA 30309
Toll-free: (800) 872-7100

Tennessee

Tennessee Chapter
Midtown Plaza
1719 West End Avenue
Suite 303-W
Nashville, TN 37203
Phone: (615)320-7626
Fax: (615)320-7399
Hours: 8:30 A.M.–4:30 P.M.
   (Central)

Texas

North Texas Chapter
2824 Swiss Avenue
Dallas, Texas 75204
Phone: (214) 826-4361
Toll-free: (800) 442-6653
Fax: (214) 824-5842
Office Hours: 8:30 A.M.–
   5:00 P.M. (Central)

Northwest Texas Chapter
3145 McCart Avenue
Fort Worth, TX 76110
Phone: (817)926-7733

South Texas Chapter
7447 Harwin
Suite 118
Houston, TX 77036
Phone: (713)785-2360
Fax: (713)785-6805
Hours: 9:00 A.M.–5:00 P.M.
   (Central)

Utah

Utah/Idaho Chapter
448 East 400 South
Suite 103
Salt Lake City, UT 84111
Phone: (801)536-0991
Hours: 8:30 A.M.–5:00 P.M.
(Mountain)

Vermont

*Northern New England
Chapter*
P.O. Box 422
257 South Union Street
Burlington, VT 05402
Phone: (802)864-4988
Fax: (802)864-5339
Hours: 8:30 A.M.–4:30 P.M.
(Eastern)

Virginia

Virginia Chapter
3805 Cutshaw Avenue,
Suite 200
Richmond, VA 23230
Tel: (804) 359-1700
Fax: (804) 359-4900
Toll-Free: (800) 456-4687
(within Virginia)
Hours: 9:00 A.M.–5:00 P.M.
(Eastern)

Washington

Washington State Chapter
100 South King, #330
Seattle, WA 98104-2864
Phone: (206)622-1378

West Virginia

Refer to the *Ohio River Valley
Chapter* or the *Maryland
Chapter*

Wisconsin

Wisconsin Chapter
8556 West National Avenue
West Allis, WI 53227
Phone: (414)321-3933

Wyoming

Serviced by:
Phone: (214) 826-4361
Toll-free: (800) 442-6653
Fax: (214) 824-5842
Office Hours: 8:30 A.M.–
5:00 P.M. (Central)

Rocky Mountain Chapter
2280 South Albion Street
Denver, Colorado 80222-
4906
Phone: (303) 756-8622
Toll-free: (800)475-6447
Fax: (303)759-4349
Hours: 8:00 A.M.–4:30 P.M.
(Mountain)

Recommended
Readings

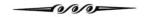

Murray, Michael, N.D. *Arthritis.* Rocklin, CA: Prima Publishing, 1994.

Pang, Chia Siew, and Goh Ewe Hock. *Tsai Chi: 10 Minutes to Health.* Sebastopol, CA: CRCS Publications, 1985.

Rothfeld, Glen S., M.D., and Susan Levert. *Natural Medicine for Arthritis.* Emmaus, PA: Rodale Press, Inc., 1996.

Washnis, George J., and Richard Z. Hricak. *Discovery of Magnetic Health: A Health Care Alternative.* Rockville, MD: Nova Publishing Company, 1993.

Bibliography

Adams, M. E., et al. "The Role of Viscosupplementation with Hylan G-F 20 (Synvisc) in the Treatment of Osteoarthritis of the Knee. A Canadian Multicentre trial comparing Hylan G-F 20 alone, Hylan G-F 20 with non-steroidal anti-inflammatory drugs (NSAID'S) and NSAID'S alone." *Osteoarthritis Cartilage*, 3 (4): 213–25, December 1995.

Ader, Robert, et al. "Psychoneuroimmunology: Interactions between the Nervous System and the Immune System (Review Article)." *The Lancet*, v. 345, n. 8942, p. 99 (5), January 14, 1995.

Andersen-Parrado, Patricia. "A Diet Rich in Omega-Three Fatty Acids and Niacinamide May Help Arthritis." *Better Nutrition*, v. 58, n. 10, p. 22 (2), October 1996.

Andersen-Parrado, Patricia. "Evidence Shows That Mom Was Right about Eating Your Broccoli." *Better Nutrition*, v. 58, n. 11, p.16 (1), November 1996.

Berger, H., et al. "Association of Radiographically Evident Osteoarthritis with Higher Bone Mineral Density and Increased Bone Loss with Edge. The Roderdam Study." *Arthritis Rheum*, 39: 1, 81–86, January 1996.

Biotech Patent News, "Gene Therapy for Arthritis Initiated at the University of Pittsburgh Medical Center." V. 10, issue 8, August 1, 1996.

Blaun, Randy. "How to Eat Smart: Foods That Benefit Brain Function." *Psychology Today*, vol. 29, n. 3, p. 34 (11), May–June 1996.

Brown, Edwin. "What You Eat Is Not Necessarily What You Get." *Medical Update*, v. 19, n. 9, p. 4 (1), March 1996.

Button, Graham. "Improvement on Copper Bracelets: Using Lasers to Treat Soft Tissue Pain." *Forbes*, vol. 144, n. 11, p. 320 (2), November 7, 1994.

Carlin, Peter, et al. "Treat the Body, Heal the Mind: Treatment of Depression." *Health*, v. 11, n. 1, p. 72 (7), January–February 1997.

Challem, Jack. "Put Out the Fire: Natural Arthritis Care." *Natural Health*, v. 27, n. 2, p. 54 (3), March–April 1997.

Cleland, K. A., et al. "Differences in Fatty Acid Composition of Immature and Mature Articular Cartilage in Humans and Sheep." *Lipids*, 30:10, 949–53, October 1995.

Clelland, Christine, et al. "Preoperative Medical Evaluation in Patients Have Joint Replacement Surgery: Added Benefits." *Medical Journal*, v. 89, n. 10, 958–60, October 1996.

Coleman, E. A., et al. "The Relationship of Joint Symptoms with Exercise Performance in Older Adults." *Journal American, Geriatric Society*, 44: 1 14–21, January 1996.

Colt, George H. "See Me, Feel Me, Touch Me, Heal Me." *Life*, September 1996, 34–50.

Corsello, Serafina, et al. "Beyond Drugs: M.D.s Use of Acupuncture, Herbs, Magnets, and Other Alternatives." *Health News and Review*, v. 4, n. 1, p. 18 (1), winter 1994.

Croft, Peter. "The Epidemiology of Pain: The More You Have, The More You Get." *Annals of the Rheumatic Diseases*, v. 55, n. 12, p. 859 (2), December 1996.

Dahlberg, Leif, et al. "Intra-articular injections of Hyaluronan in Patients with Cartilage Abnormalities and Knee Pain." *Arthritis and Rheumatism*, v. 37, 4, 521–28, April 1994.

Daltroy, L. H., et al. "Effectiveness of Minimally Supervised Home Aerobic Training in Patients with Systemic Rheumatic Disease." *British Journal of Rheumatology*, 34: 11, 1064–69, November 1995.

DeWester, Jeffrey. "Recognizing and Treating the Patient with Somatic Manifestations of Depression." *Journal of Family Practice*, v. 43, n. 6, PS 3 (13), December 1996.

Dolby, Victoria. "Shark Cartilage and Other Nutrients Make a 'Joint' Effort Against Arthritis." *Better Nutrition*, v. 58, N9, p. 32 (1), September 1996.

Dovanti, A., Bignamini, A.A., and Rovati, A.L. "Therapeutic Activity of Oral Glucosamine Sulphate in Osteoarthrosis: A

Placebo-Controlled Double-Bline Investigation." *Clinical Therapeutics* 3(4):266-272, 1980.

Dube, Loret, et al. "The Role of Emotions in Health Care Satisfaction." *The Journal of Health Care Marketing*, v. 16, n. 2, p. 45 (7), summer 1996.

Eisendrath, Stewart J. "Psychiatric Aspects of Chronic Pain." *Neurology* 45 (supplement 9): S26–S34, 1995.

Executive Healths Good Health Report, "Vitamin D Slows Progression of Arthritis of the Knee." v. 33, n. 4, p. 8 (1), January 1997.

Felson, D. T., et al. "Alcohol Intake and Bone Mineral Density in Elderly Men and Women. The Framingham Study." *American Journal Epidemiology*, 142:5, 485–92, September 1, 1995.

Felson, D. T., et al. "The Incidents and Natural History of Knee Osteoarthritis in the Elderly. The Framingham Osteoarthritis Study." *Arthritis Rheum*, 38:10, 1500–05, October 1995.

Felson, D. T. "Weight in Osteoarthritis." *American Journal of Clinical Nutrition*. 63:3 supplement, 430 S-432 S, March 1996.

Fillon, Mike. "Bloodless Surgery." *Popular Mechanics*, v. 174, n. 1, p. 48 (4), January 1997.

Fontaine, Kevin R., et al. "Health Related Quality of Life in Obese Persons Seeking Treatment." *The Journal of Family Practice*, v. 43, n. 3, 265–70, September 1996.

Food Ingredient News, "Bacterial in Food May Cause Arthritis." v. 12, issue 3, December 1, 1996. Publisher Business Communications Company, Inc.

Free, Valerie H. "Magnetic Therapy: Boosting the Body's Natural Healing." *Complimentary Healing*. P.O. Box 558, Riverside, CT 06878.

Fries, J. F., et al. "Relationship of Running to Musculoskeletal Pain with Age. A 6 year longitudinal study." *Arthritis Rheum*. 39: 1, 624–72, January 1996.

Gidrich, S. M. "Mechanisms Related to Psychological Well-Being in Older Women With Chronic Illnesses: Age and Disease Comparisons." *Res Nurs Health*, 19:3, 225–35, June 1996.

Giordano, N., et al. "The Efficacy and Safety of Glucosamine Sulfate in the Treatment of Gonarthritis." *Clin Ter*. 147 (3): 9–105.

Gowan, Kristin, et. al. "Osteoarthritis: Practical Steps to Successful Therapy." *Consultant*, v. 36, n.9, p. 2048 (6), September 1996.

Hazes, J. M. W., et al. "How Vigorously Should We Exercise Our Rheumatoid Arthritis Patients?" *Annals of Rheumatic Disease*, v. 55, n. 12, p. 861 (2), December 1996.

Health Facts, "Slow Down Osteoarthritis (with Diet Therapy)." v. 21, n. 209, p. 1 (2), October 1996 (full text copyright: 1996 Center for Medical Consumers, Inc.).

Hudnall, Marsha. "Boosting Immunity: Can Nutrition Really Make a Difference?" *Environmental Nutrition*, v. 19 and 11, p. 1 (2), November 1996.

Jamison, R. N., et al. "Weather Changes in Pain: Perceived Influence of Local Climate on Pain Complaint in Chronic Pain Patients." *Pain*, 61:2, 309–15, May 1995.

Joans, G., et al. "Osteoarthritis, Bone Density, Postural Stability, and Osteoporotic Fractures. A Population Based Study." *Journal of Rheumatology*, 22:5, 921–25, May 1995.

Jobran, Janice. "Tackle Arthritis with a Knife and Fork; New Hope That Diet Can Ease Your Pain." *Prevention*, v. 48, n. 11, p. 83 (9), November 1996.

Katzel, Leslie, et al. "Effect of Weight Loss Versus Aerobic Exercise Training on Risk Factors for Coronary Disease in Healthy, Obese, Middle-Aged and Older Men." *Journal of American Medical Association*, v. 274: 1915–21, December 27, 1995.

Kikuchit, et al. "Effect of High Molecular Weight, Hyaluronan on Cartilage." *Osteoarthritis Cartilage*, 4(2): 99–110, June 1996.

Kondziolka, Douglas, et al. "Stereotactic Radiosurgery Using the Gamma Knife: Indications and Results." *Neurologist III*, 1997: 45-52.

Lascaratos, Jay. "Arthritis in Byzantium (AD324–1453): Unknown Information from Non-Medical Literary Sources." *Rheumatologic Disease*, 54: 12, 951–57, December 1995.

Marbury, Thomas C., et al. "Placebo Controlled Dose Response Study of Dexfenfluramine in the Treatment of Obese Patients." *Current Therapeutic Research*, v. 57, n. 9, 663–74, September 1996.

Masi, A. T., et al. "Hormonal and Pregnancy Relationships to Rheumatoid Arthritis: Convergent Effects with Immunologic and Microvascular Systems." *Semin Arthritis Rheum*, 25:1, 1–27, August 1995.

McAlindon, T. E., et al. "Do Antioxidant Micronutrients Protect against the Development and Progression of Knee Osteoarthritis?" *Arthritis Rheum*, 39:4, 648–56, April 1996.

McAlindon, T. E., et al. "Relation of Dietary Intake and Serum Levels of Vitamin D to Progression of Osteoarthritis of the Knee Among Participants in the Framingham Study." *Annals of Internal Medicine*, v. 125, 353–59, September 1, 1996.

McDermott, Elizabeth, et al. "Further Evidence for Genetic Anticipation in Familial Rheumatoid Arthritis." *Annals of Rheumatic Disease*, v. 55, n. 7, p. 475 (3), July 1996.

Medical Update, "Mama's Chicken Soup Vindicated at Last? As a Remedy for Rheumatoid Arthritis." V. 17, n. 9, p. 4 (2), March 1994.

Mead, Nathaniel, et al. "Don't Drink Your Milk!" *Natural Health*, v. 24, n. 4, p. 70 (5), July–August 1994.

Messina, Mark, et al. "Foods with "Fight: Plant Foods Containing Healthful Phytochemicals." *Better Homes and Gardens*, v. 75, n. 2, p. 76 (3), February 1997.

Mitchmax, Mitchell B. "Antidepressants as Analgesics." *Pain Research and Management*, v. 1, 233–41.

Morbidity and Mortality Weekly Report, "Factors Associated with Prevalent Self-Reported Arthritis and Other Rheumatic Conditions—United States, 1989–1991." v. 45, n. 23, June 14, 1996.

Moskowitz, R. W. "The Appropriate Use of NSAID'S in Arthritic Conditions." *American Journal of Orthopedics*, v. XX5, n. 9S, 4–6, September 1996.

Müeller-Baßbender, H., et al. "Glucosamine Sulfate Compared to Ibuprofen in Osteoarthritis of the Knee." *Osteoarthritis and Cartilage* 2:61–69, 1994.

Munson, Mary. "Tank Heaven: Water Exercise May Unplug Pain." *Prevention*, v. 48, n. 11, p. 40 (2), November 1996.

Napier, Christine. "Unproven Medical Treatments, Le Elderly." *FDA Consumer*, v. 28, n. 2, p. 32 (6), March 1994.

Newton-John, Tobey R., et al. "Cognitive-Behavioral Therapy Versus EMG Biofeedback in the Treatment of Chronic Low Back Pain." *Behavior Research Theory*, v. 33, n. 6, 691–97, 1995.

Nodell, Bobby. "Magnetic Pitch Attracts Scrutiny." *Los Angeles Business Journal*, v. 15, n. 25, June 21, 1993.

Oliveria, S. A., et al. "Incidents of Symptomatic Hand, Hip, and Knee Osteoarthritis Among Patients in a Health Maintenance Organization." *Arthritis Rheum*, 38:8, 1134–41, August 1995.

Pavelka, K., Jr., et al. "Glucosamine Oglycan Polysulfuric Acid (GAGPS) in Osteoarthritis of the Knee." *Osteoarthritic Cartilage*, 3:1, 15–23, March 1995.

Peyron, J. G. "Intra-articular Hyaluronan Injections in the Treatment of Osteoarthritis: State-of-the-art Review." *General Rheumatology Supplement*, 39:10–15, August 1993.

Pipitone, V.R. "Chondroprotection with Chondroitin Sulfate." *Drugs in Experimental and Clinical Research* 17(1):3–7, 1991.

P. I.-Sunyer, Zaviar. "The NAASO Position Paper on Approval and Use of Drugs to Treat Obesity." *Obesity Research*, v. 3, n. 5, September 1995.

Raso, Jack. "Health Care Esoterica." *Nutrition Forum*, v. 12, n. 2, p. 19, (5), March–April 1995.

Rowbotham, Michael C. "Chronic Pain: From Theory to Practical Management." *Neurology* 1995; 45 (supplement 9): S5–S10.

Ruoff, Gary E. "Depression in the Patient with Chronic Pain." *General Family Practice*, v. 43, n. 6, PS 25 (10), December 1996.

Sackke "Osteoarthritis. A Continuing Challenge." *Western Journal of Medicine*, 163:6, 579–86, December, 1995.

Schiff, Michael. "A Comparison of Naprelan and Naprosyn in the Treatment of Osteoarthritis of the Knee." *American Journal of Orthopedics*, supplement, v. XX5, n. 9S, 14–20, September 1996.

Schulick, Paul. "The Healing Power of Ginger." *Vegetarian Times*, n. 225, p. 78 (4), May 1996.

Setniker, I., et al. "Antiarthritic Effects of Glucosamine Sulfate Studied in Animal Models." *Drug Res*, 41 (1):542–49, 1991.

Siegel, Lori, et al. "Viral Infection as a Cause of Arthritis." *American Family Physician*, v. 54, n. 6, p. 2009 (7), November 1, 1996.

Soldani, G. and Romagnoli, J. "Experimental and Clinical Pharmacology of Glycosaminoglycans (GAGs)." *Drugs in Experimental and Clinical Research*. 18 (1):81–85, 1991.

Spector, Tim D., et al. "Genetic Influence on Osteoarthritis in Women: A Twin Study." *British Medical Journal*, v. 312, n. 7036, p. 940 (5), April 13, 1996.

Spedding, M., et al. "Neural Control of Dieting." *Nature*, v. 380 p. 488, April 11, 1996.

Stoker, Melissa. "Non-Traditional Healing." *Orlando Business Journal*, v. 10, n. 12, August 27, 1993.

Sugimoto, H., et al. "Early Stage Rheumatoid Arthritis, Diagnostic Accuracy of MR Imaging." *Radiology*, 198:1, 185–92, January 1996.

Theodosakis, Jason, M.D., et al. *The Arthritis Cure*. NY: St. Martin's Press, 1997.

Zautra, A. J., et al. "Arthritis and Perceptions of Quality of Life: An Examination of Positive and Negative Affect in Rheumatoid Arthritis Patients." *Health Psychology*, 14:5, 399–408, September 1995.

Index

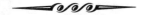

Back Pain—What Works!

A Comprehensive Guide to Preventing and Overcoming Back Problems

Joseph Kandel, M.D.
David B. Sudderth, M.D.

U.S. $14.95
Can. $19.95
ISBN 0-7615-0327-7
paperback / 224 pages

For 20 percent of all Americans, back pain is a chronic and degenerative problem that affects work, home life, and recreational activities. Here is your complete, easy-to-follow guide to understanding your back and what you can do to prevent, treat, and cure painful back problems. From preventative measures to last-resort surgery, *Back Pain—What Works!* takes the mystery out of back troubles. You'll learn all about exams, exercises, medications, surgery, alternative therapies, and much more.

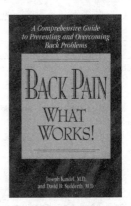

Migraine—What Works!

A Complete Guide to Overcoming and Preventing Migraines

Joseph Kandel, M.D.
David B. Sudderth, M.D.

U.S. $12.95
Can. $17.95
ISBN 0-7615-0087-1
paperback / 224 pages

Migraines are a tormenting experience for the afflicted and their families. This comprehensive handbook of medically sound solutions helps you alleviate the excruciating pain. Coauthored by two neurologists who have helped migraine sufferers for more than a decade, *Migraine—What Works!* explains in simple terms all your options for treatment and prevention. Topics covered include migraine triggers, homeopathic and pharmaceutical medicines, diet and lifestyle changes, exercises, working with physicians, and much more.

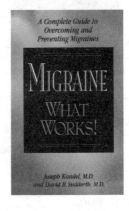

To Order Books

Please send me the following items:

Quantity	Title	Unit Price	Total
_____	_____	$ _____	$ _____
_____	_____	$ _____	$ _____
_____	_____	$ _____	$ _____
_____	_____	$ _____	$ _____
_____	_____	$ _____	$ _____

Shipping and Handling depend on Subtotal.

Subtotal	Shipping/Handling
$0.00–$14.99	$3.00
$15.00–$29.99	$4.00
$30.00–$49.99	$6.00
$50.00–$99.99	$10.00
$100.00–$199.99	$13.50
$200.00+	Call for Quote

Foreign and all Priority Request orders:
Call Order Entry department
for price quote at 916/632-4400

This chart represents the total retail price of books only (before applicable discounts are taken).

Subtotal $ _____

Deduct 10% when ordering 3-5 books $ _____

7.25% Sales Tax (CA only) $ _____

8.25% Sales Tax (TN only) $ _____

5.0% Sales Tax (MD and IN only) $ _____

Shipping and Handling* $ _____

Total Order $ _____

By Telephone: With MC or Visa, call 800-632-8676 or 916-632-4400.
Mon–Fri, 8:30-4:30.
WWW: http://www.primapublishing.com

By Internet E-mail: sales@primapub.com

By Mail: Just fill out the information below and send with your remittance to:

**Prima Publishing
P.O. Box 1260BK
Rocklin, CA 95677**

My name is _____

I live at _____

City _____ State _____ ZIP_____

MC/Visa#_____ Exp. _____

Check/money order enclosed for $ _____ Payable to Prima Publishing

Daytime telephone _____

Signature _____